Carte Weaver
2/27/2019   1.⁰⁰

The
Brain
Chemistry
Diet

Also by Michael Lesser, M.D.
Nutrition and Vitamin Therapy

MICHAEL LESSER, M.D.

with Colleen Kapklein

The Brain Chemistry Diet

The Personalized Prescription for Balancing Mood,
Relieving Stress, and Conquering Depression,
Based on Your Personality Profile

G. P. PUTNAM'S SONS
NEW YORK

Every effort has been made to ensure that the information contained in this book is complete and accurate. However, neither the publisher nor the author is engaged in rendering professional advice or services to the individual reader. The ideas, procedures, and suggestions contained in this book are not intended as a substitute for consulting with your physician and obtaining medical supervision as to any activity, procedure, or suggestion that might affect your health. Accordingly, individual readers must assume responsibility for their own actions, safety, and health, and neither the author nor the publisher shall be liable or responsible for any loss, injury, or damage allegedly arising from any information or suggestion in this book. The opinions expressed in this book represent the personal views of the author and not of the publisher.

This book, while based on true incidents, is not meant to betray any professional or personal confidences. Therefore, the author has taken the liberty of changing all of the names and identifying characteristics of the patients, doctors, nurses, staff, sites, and situations described in order to protect the privacy of those involved.

G. P. Putnam's Sons
Publishers Since 1838
a member of
Penguin Putnam Inc.
375 Hudson Street
New York, NY 10014

Copyright © 2002 by Michael Lesser, M.D., with Colleen Kapklein
All rights reserved. This book, or parts thereof, may not
be reproduced in any form without permission.
Published simultaneously in Canada

Library of Congress Cataloging-in-Publication Data

Lesser, Michael.
The brain chemistry diet : the personalized prescription for balancing
mood, relieving stress, and conquering depression, based on your
personality profile / Michael Lesser, with Colleen Kapklein.
p. cm.
Includes index.
ISBN 0-399-14744-6
1. Neurochemistry.   2. Neuropsychology.   3. Personality—
Nutritional aspects.   4. Orthomolecular therapy.   5. Dietary supplements.   6. Depression, Mental—Nutritional aspects.
I. Kapklein, Colleen.   II. Title.
QP356.3 .L47 2002   2001048358
612.8'042—dc21

Printed in the United States of America
1   3   5   7   9   10   8   6   4   2

This book is printed on acid-free paper. ∞

BOOK DESIGN BY TANYA MAIBORODA

And by the stream upon its bank . . .
shall grow all trees for food. . . .
It shall bring forth new fruit every month . . .
because their waters have issued out of
the sanctuary, and its fruit shall be for
food, and its leaf for medicine.

EZEKIEL 47:12

The Jerusalem Bible

Acknowledgments

First, I humbly acknowledge the Lord G-D Almighty, King of the Universe, from whom all blessings flow: may He bless this book and the uses made of it.

My special appreciation to my editor, Jeremy Katz; my agent, Janis Vallely; writer Henry Dreher; Washington psychiatrist James Gordon, M.D.; and especially Colleen Kapklein, for the vital roles they all played in begetting *The Brain Chemistry Diet*.

Sincerest thanks to my family: my wife, Deborah; my brothers, Laurence and Martin; and my children, Elijah, Rebecca, Sarah, and Hannah Lesser for their invaluable advice and assistance.

Certainly, I acknowledge my patients, from whom I've gained most of my practical knowledge of therapy. "Listen to your patients," said the late, great Dr. Walter Alvarez; "Listen and they will tell you what's wrong with them. And if you listen long enough, they will even tell you what will make them well."

Let me pay tribute to the new science of orthomolecular medicine, which made it possible to write this book. The legendary psychiatrist Sigmund Freud originally tried to map our character on the brain before abandoning the effort as "premature." Today, with the advances of molecular chemistry, it's possible to attempt something akin to Freud's dream.

I gratefully acknowledge the early pioneers: practitioners Abram Hoffer, M.D., Ph.D., of Victoria, B.C., Canada; Humphry Osmond, M.D., of Appleton, Wisconsin; Carl C. Pfeiffer, M.D.*; David Hawkins, M.D., of Sidona, Arizona; José A. Yar-Yura Tobias, M.D., of Great Neck, New York; Frederick Klenner, M.D.*; Emmanuel "Cherry" Cheraskin, D.D.S.*; Ben Feingold, M.D.*; Walter Alvarez, M.D.*; Thoren Randolph, M.D.*; Allen Cott, M.D.*; Harvey Ross, M.D.*; Carl Reich, M.D.*; Max Gerson, M.D.* I also thank such scientists as Linus Pauling, Ph.D.* and Roger Williams, Ph.D.*, and writers like Adele Davis* and Carlton Fredericks, Ph.D.

Thanks to my contemporaries: Hyla Cass, M.D., of Pacific Palisades, California; Priscilla Slagle, M.D., of Palm Springs, California; Bernard Rimland, Ph.D., of San Diego, California; Richard Kunin, M.D., of San Francisco, California; Michael Schachter, M.D., of Suffern, New York; Gary Null, Ph.D., of New York City; Gary Vickar, M.D., of St. Louis, Missouri; Serafina Corsello, M.D., of New York City; Eric R. Braverman, M.D., of New York City; Hugh D. Riordan, M.D., of Wichita, Kansas; Parriss M. Kidd, Ph.D., of El Cerrito, California.

I'm proud of great colleagues in other medical disciplines, but space doesn't allow. So thanks, and I'm grateful that there are now so many as to make it impossible to list them all.

ISAAC LOUIS MICHAEL LESSER, M.D.

*deceased

Contents

Foreword

You will observe with concern how long a useful truth may be known and exist, before it is generally received and practiced on.

—BENJAMIN FRANKLIN

I am delighted that Dr. Lesser has added one more to the many fine books that provide the public with the latest information about using the best diet and nutritional supplements for maintaining good health and fighting disease. For although others have gone this road before (although never in exactly this way), as Franklin noted, sometimes it takes quite a while for the message to really get through. To help you understand Dr. Lesser's achievement and appreciate it as I do, you should understand a bit about the historical struggle that preceded it. The underlying idea—using natural molecules that are commonly present in the body, in optimum doses, aimed at correcting nutrient imbalances in the body (what we call orthomolecular medicine) may seem straightforward enough. But unfortunately, straightforward is not always what is prized in modern medicine.

That's too bad, because orthomolecular medicine, besides being gentle and natural, also gets good results. It *works*. Even conditions against which modern medicine (including preventive medicine and mental health) has had much less success than it has had against simple diseases (such as bacterial infections) respond well to this new form of nutritional medicine. It is a seemingly simple, yet profoundly effective, approach.

Orthomolecular medicine, as it has developed over the past forty years, represents a major paradigm shift, so, not surprisingly, widespread acceptance in the mainstream medical world has been slow. Even as far as nutritional medicine is concerned, orthomolecular medicine is a radically different way of viewing the world. Let's call it the third wave.

The first wave was, for thousands of years, the only useful model of medicine: Through experience and observation, humans knew that certain foods and non-food plants made people sick, while others helped them heal. (Some cultures even learned that some ways of preparing food were healthier than others. For instance, Indians in Central America long ago discovered that soaking ground corn in alkali essentially ended their corn-based diet's association with pellagra. In another era, modern nutritionists would discover that pellagra is basically niacin deficiency; while early Central Americans couldn't have put it that way, their technique, it turns out, worked because soaking the corn that way releases the corn's niacin, making it available to the body.)

You can hear echoes of this ancient first-wave approach even today: As long as you eat enough food, you'll get everything your body needs. Of course, there was no other option back then.

And so it was for the majority of human medical history. It wasn't until biochemists were able to break food into its major and minor component parts (carbohydrates, protein, amino acids, fat, vitamins and minerals) that this way of thinking could be challenged. Once that occurred, the second wave emerged. This second wave focused on vitamins as preventers of disease.

By the end of the nineteenth century, there was evidence that processed foods could not maintain health even when they contained ample amounts of the three major calorie providers (carbohydrates, protein, and fat). Dr.

Casimir Funk coined the word *vitamin* in the early 1900s, though the first specific vitamin (vitamin A) wasn't identified until 1915.

But there was tremendous resistance to the new idea that foods contain accessory factors that were required for good health. At that time, the golden age of bacteriology was capturing the imagination of the medical world. With the understanding of bacteria as disease-causing contaminants, the popular belief was that the ultimate source of all disease had been found. No attention was paid to the idea that disease might be the result of a deficiency of something. So unreceptive was the medical profession that, for example, the doctor who discovered vitamin A was forced to promote his achievement by means of public lectures and articles in the mainstream (not medical) press.

Still, the second wave picked up steam, and by 1945, the majority of vitamins had been isolated. They had also been synthesized, so it became possible to add specific nutrients to your daily diet. All vitamins were found to be extraordinarily safe, closer in safety to food than to the many chemicals used in medicines. But their main use was in nearly across-the-board prevention of the major vitamin deficiency diseases, including beriberi, scurvy, and rickets as well as pellagra.

Thus the vitamins-as-prevention paradigm eventually won the field, predicated on the notions that (1) supplements are needed only to replace the few nutrients that are lacking in the diet, and when the diet is good, no supplements are needed; (2) vitamins are needed only in very small amounts to prevent deficiency diseases; (3) there was no other reason to use vitamins except regarding deficiency diseases; and (4) beyond that, taking vitamins was wasteful and did nothing more than give you vitamin-rich urine.

This turned out to be an extremely powerful position, and it still holds sway in most quarters today. However, the production of vitamins in pure, relatively inexpensive form carried within it the seeds for the next wave, as forward-thinking physicians began experimenting with them on their patients—and on themselves. The medical literature between 1930 and 1940 is rich with clinical accounts of how large doses of vitamins were helpful in treating diseases not considered to be vitamin-deficiency diseases.

Not all progress came happily or easily, however. For example, Canadian Drs. Evan and Shute were ostracized and labeled quacks for their work, which included pioneering studies in using large doses of vitamin E in patients with heart disease. (Fifty years later, they have been fully vindicated by the recent studies proving that vitamin E supplements decrease heart attacks by up to 50 percent.) I caught plenty of flack myself for my work with Dr. Humphrey Osmond on using large doses of niacin for treatment of schizophrenia, even though we were the first psychiatrists to use double-blind controlled trials, which are now the "gold standard" of medical research. Along the way, we discovered that significant doses of niacin could lower cholesterol levels, another finding that by now has been well established.

In fact, niacin was the first vitamin to be accepted by the FDA for lowering cholesterol levels. That insight notwithstanding, the FDA is a leading opponent of this kind of third-wave—orthomolecular—medicine, where vitamins are considered therapeutic. The old way is very well defended, not only by the FDA but also by the medical establishment, medical schools, medical journals, nutritionists, government agencies, and the food industry.

Even in the face of such opposition, after thirty-five years of slow accumulation of interest and data, the third wave has developed especially rapidly over the past five years. It is built around four parameters: (1) Even the best diet will not be adequate for a large proportion of the population, especially people under psychological or physiological stress, and optimum diets are rare and becoming increasingly difficult to obtain anyway; (2) Vitamin supplements are needed in optimum amounts, which may be either large or small, depending on the nature and severity of the stress; (3) Many non-deficiency diseases respond to optimum doses of vitamins, and even more are being discovered as research expands; and (4) The best medicine consists of the proper use of nutrient supplements along with the best complete diet.

This is the torch that Dr. Lesser picks up. Actually, he's been carrying it for decades. But as I mentioned, there are already many books covering the subject. Why then do we need yet another one, even one as good as this one? Well, apart from the facts that every new book captures a new and different audience and that this book focuses on mental health in particular, Dr. Lesser's unique contribution is his use of sophisticated clinical profiles of patients as the basis of his therapeutic program, which provides a unique way of determining what is best for your body.

The attempt to categorize patients into types is not new. It was done perhaps most famously by Carl Jung, and Jungian therapists still use his personality types today. Modern psychiatry has taken categorizing to ridiculous extremes, however, and huge tomes are now required to keep track of the numerous diagnostic codes. That is definitely not what Dr. Lesser is doing here. Rather, he is providing an antidote to that rampant extremism. His system, both simple and profound on its own, also improves the results of treatment by eliminating much of the trial and error that has often been necessary.

He divides people into six basic brain types. Each is described in detail, and precise instructions on how to identify your own type are given, along with information on the foods you should consume (and avoid), and the nutrients, vitamins, minerals, fatty acids, and even herbs that in his experience work best for that particular type. He also includes guidance on the best laboratory tests, since even the best clinician cannot (and should not) depend solely upon clinical judgment when objective tests are available. Dr. Lesser advises using all the information available—observational, orthomolecular, clinical, laboratory, experiential—in arriving at a brain type and in choosing therapies accordingly. I urge readers to study his system of brain types as seriously as he has, and to try this approach and discover for themselves its great potential.

Dr. Lesser is one of the pioneers in the development of orthomolecular psychiatry and medicine, and this book represents a very serious attempt by a very experienced physician to provide a rational system of diagnosis and treatment to make therapies already available much more effective. I don't know if this typology will be useful in deciding which drugs should be used; I rather doubt it. But this does not matter since in orthomolecular psychiatry, although we take advantage of the best that modern medicine has to offer, drugs take a much lesser role. They are crutches to be used in a crisis and then discarded as soon as possible to allow your body to maintain its strength. They certainly are not the be-all and end-all of treatment, as the drug companies would have you believe.

Best of all, in my opinion, is the last chapter, The Brain Chemistry Diet, which provides a very good, succinct account of the optimum diet. While no one diet is a panacea—the best diet is always one tailored to the individual—Dr. Lesser provides six key commandments (my term): (1) Eat a rich variety of natural foods; (2) Choose fresh, whole foods that are as close as possible to their natural state; (3) Opt for clean foods, using organic and free-range items whenever possible; (4) Get a good amount of healthy fats and oils, but strictly limit saturated fats and trans-fatty acids; (5) Complement an imperfect diet with nutritional supplements; and (6) Remember that how you eat is as important as what you eat. This is a very useful addition to the clinical nutritional literature all by itself.

—A. HOFFER, M.D., PH.D., FRCP(C)
September 25, 2001

Sarah, Brain Chemistry, and Me

The way Sarah walked into my office, leading an entourage of family members that included her husband, father, mother, and siblings, it took me a minute to identify her as the woman who had called me for help. Even though Sarah was the one in distress, her charisma made her stand out like a shining star at the center of the group. Despite her problems, Sarah saw the situation more clearly than anybody else could. She had a definite agenda and came in that day to get it solved. Like everything else, she would take therapy into her own hands. The rest of us were merely her assistants.

Sarah's vibrance and intensity were quite a counterpoint to her tale of woe. Sarah said she was tearful all the time and constantly fatigued. She told me she felt impatient, irritable, and anxious. She felt as if she had to face each day with no energy, forcing herself to be "up."

"It's like I have to think hard to remember my old charming self, and then act out being me," Sarah confided.

Since taking the antidepressant her internist prescribed, her crying jags were less frequent, but she complained that the side effects made her feel like some kind of automaton, as if she were running on automatic pilot. And the medicine gave her headaches and nausea.

Sarah had suffered through six miscarriages and still hadn't completed a healthy pregnancy. She and her husband certainly seemed to be deeply in love, and those in her extended family of parents and siblings were as supportive of her as she was devoted to them, so I saw no obvious psychological reason for the multiple miscarriages. Her mother, grandmother, aunts, and sisters had many uneventful pregnancies between them, so the miscarriages didn't seem to be genetically linked either.

It was clear that Sarah was a strong person, able to grow because of what she'd been through, rather than wallowing in it. But she talked about the parts of her she felt were missing. The single most distressing thing to her was that either the drugs or the underlying depression was robbing her of her creativity. A talented artist—one who made a living with her painting—she used to jump up every morning anxious to get started on her creations. Now she couldn't remember the last time she had any interest in working on a canvas.

Furthermore, though Sarah was in her early thirties, her sex drive had disappeared years ago and still hadn't returned even with the medication. She told me she no longer even had dreams of a sexual nature. She also worried that her memory was not as strong as it once was.

"It's just too hard to stay happy when this happens over and over again," Sarah said.

It was my reputation as a nutritional doctor and a psychiatrist that landed Sarah in my office. She asked me to help her get off the prescription antidepressants, so that she could try again to carry a pregnancy to term and not expose the fetus to a risk of birth defects. But she was worried that she would really bottom out without the pills. She also wanted me to help her body handle a full-term pregnancy, and help her manage the stress of getting and being pregnant when her past experiences had been so grim.

Unlike most doctors who would speculate about whether her depression might be contributing to the problem pregnancies or if the problem pregnancies might be causing her depression, I didn't much care which way it worked. No doubt the relationship between the two problems was complicated. More important still than the specific causes were the possible solutions. Sarah had been through talk therapy, and she'd tried drug therapy, but neither had worked.

With Sarah, as with most of my patients, I didn't believe the answer lay in either of these areas. As always, I first considered the physical functioning of her body, both the underlying biochemistry and the overall quality of nutrition. Although it may be hard to believe, malnutrition is a severe epidemic in this country, and I knew that proper nutrition was going to be Sarah's most powerful weapon.

From decades of working with people struggling with everything from grief, to work stress, to minor neuroses, to schizophrenia, to psychosis, to major antisocial behavior, I'd learned gentle, natural, and—most of all—effective ways to rebalance the brain's chemistry, stabilizing moods while reducing and often eliminating the need for synthetic drugs. In Sarah's case, this meant giving her vitamin E, bioflavonoids, and folic acid to help prevent miscarriage; copper to address her deficiency; a diet to counteract low blood sugar; and a B-complex vitamin to fight depression. That's all she needed to wean herself off medication, to rediscover her regular, cheerful, optimistic, creative self, and to prepare her body for motherhood.

Prescription drugs have their place and purpose. But they are harsh, sometimes toxic, and often addictive, and must be used with great care, despite the current tendency to almost casually recommend and use these chemicals. Furthermore, drugs treat symptoms, but not the root of the problem. The nutritional treatments that I've learned over the years can provide all the benefits of prescription drugs with none of the risks for anyone willing to work a little harder than taking a supposed "magic bullet" requires. They also complement—and sometimes replace—talk therapies. Talk certainly has its place, too, but it can be expensive and time-consuming. And some people just aren't emotionally wired to make use of it.

But we all eat, and we all make choices about what we eat. My preference is always for the natural, safe, and effective nutritional approach rather than the riskier use of prescription drugs. So I recommend a diet tailored to an individual's particular brain chemistry. I always recommend some supplements of vitamins and minerals. I usually prescribe relatively large doses because I am using the vitamins like a prescription drug. To get the drug effect and overcome deficiencies and chronic malnutrition, a large dose is necessary. I also often use amino acids, enzymes, fatty acids, and herbs, depending on the specific case.

I'm an eclectic doctor—I use what works. So I write out prescriptions for Prozac, lithium, and other drugs on the few occasions when they fill the bill. But I look on those as only temporary interventions, at best, and I prefer gentler methods. No treatment is without risk, and "natural" does not necessarily mean "safe." Cobra venom, for example, is natural, and even beneficial herbs like ephedra have been proven to have very real dangers associated with them. You have to consider the risk/benefit ratio for any treatment—and for living without treatment.

For Sarah, drug treatment was apparently an improvement over no treatment. But she was missing the even greater benefits that natural substances can bring, while suffering from some of the common side effects from drugs. Still, she feared what she would face if she were to simply stop taking her medication—and rightly so. Fortunately, a complete physical revealed that a few simple diet and supplement solutions were possible.

A five-hour glucose tolerance test revealed that Sarah had severe hypoglycemia—low blood sugar—which often manifests as depression. Her copper levels were also below normal, which can often result in fatigue and may be linked to infertility. Her zinc levels were actually higher than normal. That alone wouldn't usually be a problem, but the balance between copper and zinc is crucial—and delicate. Therefore, a high zinc level combined with a low copper level would exacerbate the problems of not having enough copper.

All the other vitamins and nutrients were within normal ranges. "Normal" doesn't necessarily mean "optimal," however, or even fully functional, so I recommended that she take vitamin E, bioflavonoids, and folic acid anyway, as they all are crucial for healthy pregnancies and for helping to prevent miscarriages. I also recommended that she take a B-complex vitamin, particularly for the niacin and thiamine, which I've found to be particularly helpful for weepy depressions. And, of course, I recommended copper to correct her low levels of the mineral.

The most important advice I gave Sarah was to follow a diet designed to control her hypoglycemia, evening out her blood sugar levels and avoiding steep peaks and sharp drops: a basically healthy lowfat diet, but with relatively high amounts of protein. I recommended that she strictly avoid white sugar, white flour, and white rice, and minimize stimulants, such as caffeine and alcohol. I also stressed that she eat small, frequent meals centered on whole, fresh, unrefined foods. Any time she felt herself thinking unpleasant—depressed—thoughts, she learned to make the association, "Oh, my blood sugar is low," and would have a small high-protein snack.

Finally, I gave Sarah guidelines on how to gradually reduce the dose of the antidepressant she was taking.

Two and a half months later, Sarah came to my office for her third visit, and this time a fully alive and energetic woman sat across from me, smiling. "I barely recognize the person I used to be," she told me. "I don't have to force this cheerful front anymore. It is *me* now. My old self is back again."

Sarah was back at her easel with gusto and had given me one of her new paintings as a gift. It depicted two horses splashing along a sun-drenched beach, as joyful an image as I've ever seen. I needed no further proof of her improvement.

Thanks to her new diet and supplements, within one month all her symptoms had disappeared. Her energy had returned and her mood had stabilized. She'd obviously rediscovered her creativity, and she said her sex drive was also back in full force. Her crying jags had completely stopped. She'd stopped feeling nervous all the time. She was no longer snapping at her husband for no reason or making her family miserable. Her days living like death warmed over were finished.

"I would never have dreamed the way I was eating was making me feel so lousy," she said.

After the first month on the new program, Sarah had slowly weaned herself off the antidepressants. She suffered no withdrawal symptoms and did not slide back into depression. She was so pleased with her progress, she announced that she and her husband were ready to try to conceive again.

When human beings are functioning smoothly—when they are properly nourished and not under any other unusual stress—they feel good. They are optimistic. They know that being alive is a wonderful thing. Sarah had nearly lost sight of that until a simple rebalancing of her brain chemistry restored the gift of that knowledge.

In most cases, as in Sarah's, problems—even those that loom the largest—are only the result of a flawed outlook on life. That outlook, in turn, is the result of faulty chemistry. The bad news is how easily the chemistry is thrown out of balance in our hectic modern lives. But the good news is that we have a host of simple, natural, gentle strategies that can bring us back on track.

I didn't hear from Sarah again until a year and a half later, when she called to announce that she'd given birth a few months earlier. She'd had a healthy pregnancy and delivery, and her depressive symptoms had not returned. She still took her vitamins, though she'd relaxed her diet somewhat once she felt her blood sugar levels had stabilized. She knew a little something more about fatigue, now, waking up to nurse her son every few hours through the night, but sounded gleeful as she described it.

With that, Sarah walked out of my life for years. Then, one fall afternoon, I answered the phone and found to my surprise that it was Sarah's father. He had a problem of his own and remembered how I'd helped his daughter. I recommended a colleague in his area but not before he gave me an update on Sarah. She's now a mother of four, and he told me that the family was grateful to have the "real" Sarah back. They'd been at the end of their rope trying to help her before she came to see me.

Depression and other mood disorders caused by biochemical imbalances can be literally life threatening. Much more commonly, however, as in Sarah's case, they steal the ease and joy out of life. What's shocking is how often that happens as a result of malnutrition—and how often the simple yet powerful remedies that can correct the situation are overlooked. One half of my mission in this book is to make you aware of the nutritional treatments that can help you balance your own brain chemistry, establishing optimal moods. (We'll get to the other half a bit later in this chapter.)

Ironically, in this relatively wealthy modern society, our diets are so deficient in crucial nutrients and so overloaded with sugars and other artificial and short-acting stimulants that many people are actually suffering from malnourishment. Poor nutrition can render our body chemistry so out of whack that depression or other mood disorders result even without the external factors—a job from hell or a foundering marriage—that we generally tend to blame.

Those factors can definitely contribute to a bad situation, and they are much more likely to happen to malnourished people. When we are healthy, we make better choices in jobs and mates, for example—and attract better options. The whole thing is circular: Being malnourished makes it more likely that you are miserable at your job or are involved in a miserable relationship. If you're miserable, you're more likely to go home after work and try to erase the day with a couple of beers, some sweet, fatty "treats," or by vegetating in front of the television—which will make you (or keep you) malnourished. You can hop on this train at any point in the cycle, but getting off takes a bit of work.

The body needs proper nourishment to function physically, mentally, and emotionally. Without proper nutrition, we can't handle the many stresses we all face. The dynamic balance of chemicals within our brains goes haywire, and what we label anxiety, depression, and obsession, among many other unpleasant things in a variety of intensities, result.

I didn't learn much about nutrition in medical school. In pharmacology, only one day's lecture was devoted to vitamins, while we spent several months on various types of drugs. Vitamins were regarded as a bit of physiology you needed to stay alive, and vitamin deficiency was considered to be a cause of disease—but extremely rare. Like high school biology students everywhere, we learned that vitamin C was discovered when sailors who were at sea for months at a time without any fresh food developed scurvy (weakness, wasting, anemia, swelling, and bleeding) and recovered by sucking on limes, which are rich in vitamin C. To this day, the recommended daily allowance of vitamin C is basically the amount you need *not* to get scurvy. I got to wondering if this wasn't a sad underestimation of the potential power of this and all nutrients.

It wasn't until years later that I ran across another classic story from the annals of mental health medicine that sealed my conviction that giving short shrift to nutrition meant providing second-class health care. In the early part of this century, more than 200,000 people in this country had pellagra, and many of them were institutionalized. Gruesome physical symptoms (gastrointestinal disturbances and scabs and oozing sores all over the body) accompanied the "nervous" disorders that landed victims in mental hospitals. Locking them up also served to quarantine them, as pellagra was originally thought to be viral and infectious, and was often fatal.

Then, a senior United States Public Health Service officer assigned to the problem, Dr. Joseph D. Goldberger, wondered why pellagra was much more common in rural areas of the South. He also wondered why the staff in these institutions never caught this supposedly infectious disease. When he noticed that the staff and patients had separate menus, he guessed that diet might play an important role. Lo and behold, when he added meats, vegetables, and milk to the extremely low-quality meals the patients lived on, these "crazy" people had dramatic recoveries. Their sores dried up and disappeared, their stomachs settled down, and they no longer appeared insane in the least.

Research showed that pellagra is a deficiency in niacin (vitamin B3). Even before they came to the mental hospitals, the patients lived in very poor areas that yielded a very poor diet. Many of them were subsisting on little more than corn and refined cornmeal, and so they were not getting the full range of nutrients the body needs. The food in the hospital was of no higher quality, yet simple sound nutrition was all they needed. In the wake of the acceptance of his theories, 100,000 people were discharged from hospitals across the American South, well nourished—and cured.

This amazing story about the power of nutrients certainly wasn't the sort of thing we discussed in medical school. Most of what I learned, even decades ago, was focused on high technology and elaborate pharmacology. Impressive new drugs were constantly being developed, and things once thought of as the province of science fiction were becoming reality—like organ transplants. As miraculous as many of these new things were, we all seemed to be expected to have blind faith in them, and they eclipsed older wisdom about the body and the ways it functioned best. We were crammed full of information about disease but learned surprisingly little about health.

After medical school, during internship and psychiatry residence, there was more of an ongoing and obvious conflict between high- and low-tech methods. But here it was the newer medical model—centered on pharmacology—versus the classic Freudian analytical model. Talk therapy was already losing ground in the face of new drugs that seemed to come out of top labs almost every month. As scientists discovered the biological roots of mental and emotional ailments, and zeroed in on maintaining healthy chemical balances in the brain, the solutions were always assumed to be drugs.

I was wowed by the ability of some of these powerful drugs to completely change a person's behavior, as well as their sometimes alarming side effects. Gradually I began to wonder if there might not be natural ways to affect the chemicals that do, after all, appear naturally in the body, *without* bringing out these big guns.

Mainly, however, I was busy soaking up all I could from the doctors mentoring me. My internship year (the first year out of medical school, when you're finally doing clinical medicine full time), I worked under Thomas Szasz, who made "the myth of mental illness" a famous phrase. I also heard a series of lectures by the Scottish psychiatrist R. D. Laing, who viewed insanity as a valid voyage of personal discovery. Social problems might be to blame, they both allowed. In any case, talk therapy was the primary solution—if a "solution" was needed at all. If there is no problem (only a "myth" or self-discovery), there's no need for a solution. Talk therapy, then, would just be a completely optional way to enhance what you learn about yourself.

The next year, residency put me in a totally different environment, in a hospital where mental illness was viewed as a permanent, genetic disease—something you most certainly could not talk your way out of. Tranquilizers were the most popular treatment. The drugs we were using then were much rougher than what we have today, but at the time, they were the latest word in psychiatry.

As I was steeped in each of these attitudes in turn, I embraced the arguments of the people I was working most closely with at the time. But when the time came to go out on my own, I realized I had to figure out what *I* believed. I needed to settle on the approach I would take with my own patients. And I realized that I didn't fully connect with anything I had been exposed to thus far. I wasn't ready to whip out the prescription pad for every person who walked through my door, but I didn't want to throw that pad out, either. I liked the objectivity of prescribing a specific dose of a specific medicine for a specific illness. I also knew that talking with patients was helping a lot of them, though not everyone benefited. For those that did, it often took a long, long time.

Fortunately for me, the year I finished my residency, Nobel Prize–winning chemist Linus Pauling published an article in *Science* that revolutionized my outlook. In it, he coined the term "orthomolecular" psychiatry, renaming what had been generally referred to (by the few who cared to discuss it) as megavitamin therapy. "Ortho" is from the Greek, meaning right or straight or correct (as in "orthodox" and "orthodontist"). Pauling saw both treatment of illness and prevention of disease as a matter of successfully varying the concentrations in the body of substances normally present in the body: the right molecules in the right amounts.

"The functioning of the brain is affected by the molecular concentrations of many substances that are normally present in the brain," he wrote. But "the optimum concentrations of these substances for a person may differ greatly from the concentrations provided by his normal diet and genetic machinery." If your body isn't making or handling the key substances well, and your diet most likely isn't making up for it, you need individually tailored nutritional supplements to correct the imbalance.

Pauling's emphasis was on vitamins and minerals, though the field has since expanded to include amino acids, enzymes, botanical medicines, fatty acids, and other nutrients. The field has also since branched out from psychiatry to include all aspects of medicine. The main idea has stayed the same: to provide the same benefits that drugs do, but with natural sub-stances instead of prescription medications, or in addition to greatly re-duced doses. "Natural" solutions are intuitively appealing to a lot of people, including me, but there's also a very real plus in avoiding the sometimes heavy-duty side effects that heavy-duty drugs often bring with them.

Pauling's article made quite a splash. Here was a two-time winner of the Nobel Prize, a world-famous chemist, speaking out on the importance of *vitamins*. Some people on the fringe had been talking them up, but those people always seemed to be selling pipe dreams and saying not to worry about the scientific evidence backing up their medical claims. For the first time, someone the general public—and the scientific and medical commu-nities—trusted was saying that what we'd been hearing from a few lonely voices was worth listening to after all.

It was Peter, a "chronic schizophrenic," who taught me that mental illness is *not* a myth. The label is surely unnecessary and limiting, but Peter had a very real problem and was seeking a very real answer. So, electrified by the promise of Pauling's position, I did more research and discovered that the first ever double-blind study (science's "gold standard") of schizophrenia in North America focused on nutrition. A series of clinical trials by Drs. Abram Hoffer and Humphrey Osmond in Canada in the 1950s showed that, compared to patients given a placebo or electroshock therapy, patients treated with niacin only were more likely to function successfully, more likely to be rid of symptoms entirely, more likely to remain well five years after the treatment, and *less* likely to land back in the hospital again.

If nothing more than a short-term dose of a B vitamin could restore a person with chronic schizophrenia to normal, I could not understand why this work was so soon forgotten by mainstream medicine. I was determined to get Peter to try it. Worst-case scenario, I knew, was that this would join a long line of failed approaches. It certainly could do no harm. So I consulted with the best minds available: Drs. Hoffer and Osmond, as well as another pioneer in this field, Dr. Carl C. Pfeiffer. Dr. Pfeiffer took on Peter as a pa-tient, and prescribed zinc, niacin, and a high-protein diet. Under doctor's orders, Peter also gave up caffeine and cigarettes.

Within three months, he was a changed person. He was calm and interactive, no longer bizarre and autistic. You could hold an actual conversation with him. He showed interest in the world around him. He became a contributing member of his family. He still wasn't a nine-to-five type, but then most "schizophrenics" probably never will be. But now that he was no longer emotionally troubled, he was able to work every day in the family business.

This was the first thing that ever helped Peter, and it has continued working for years and years. And it was the first time I personally witnessed the potency of a nutritional cure. I was sold. If taking the right vitamins and eating the right foods could heal even the sickest individuals—when sometimes it is the only thing that will help at all—just imagine what it could do for a person with garden-variety stresses! This was surely powerful stuff.

Within a couple of years, the Academy of Orthomolecular Psychiatry (now defunct; currently, the International Society of Orthomolecular Medicine carries the torch) was formed, and I was a member almost from the beginning. A simple premise held the organization together: What you eat can affect the way you think and act. For someone trained in traditional medicine, that premise sometimes seemed really unorthodox, no matter how simple it actually was, and I got used to mainstream psychiatry labeling orthomolecular practitioners as quacks and charlatans. But I never had to look further than the obvious examples of my next cup of coffee or glass of wine to be reminded of the power that the foods we ingest have on our bodies and brains.

In my eight years in official medical training, I may not have gotten much experience with nutrition, but I did spend plenty of time talking to and getting to know people with all kinds of "psychiatric problems." My internship and residency working primarily with inpatients, and my stints working in a prison and a rehab center, exposed me to many of the sickest patients. I logged a lot of hours with psychotic and schizophrenic people, and people so severely depressed that they needed to be hospitalized. I treated people completely paralyzed by anxiety and phobias, and incapacitated by obsessive-compulsive disorders or addictions. I worked with people with out-of-control manic depression, as well as full-blown sociopaths.

It was working with these extremes, surprisingly, that I learned the most about everyday people with ordinary behavior. At first, these people seemed as foreign to me as aliens, and their conditions scared me as much as the most horrible death. In fact, it often seemed to be as if they were the walking dead. Still, I couldn't help but see the human side of these people. I was personally motivated to try to make sense out of the patients.

I eventually realized that mental illness is not just something from another planet. The things we all have in common are greater than the differences. The patients I was seeing weren't just some people who were genetically misfortunate. I began to think that anybody might be crazy or sane, under the right kind of stress.

As a volunteer at a free clinic in Los Angeles, I worked with a very specific type of "crazy" people: hippies on bad trips. Some of them were suffering from serious psychosis, but we knew it wasn't because of how their mothers treated them, or because they had a bit of bad luck with the gene pool, or because they were poor. We knew their behavior was caused by drugs. That was a breakthrough insight for me: This behavior was chemical related. It became clear to me that any substance that monkeyed with the chemicals in the brain could cause a dramatic reaction. It didn't have to be deeply disturbed behavior caused by LSD overdose—it could also be depression or anxiety caused by caffeine or undernourishment.

Working with addicts—heroin being the drug of choice where I worked—also set me to thinking about addiction problems, and I realized almost all of us are addicted to something. Coffee addiction, for one, is shared by probably 90 percent of the adult American population. Even if coffee or some other source of caffeine isn't your bag, think about sugar, alcohol, chocolate, or just plain overeating. There are better and worse things to be addicted to, to be sure, but the underlying need is the same. I worked with some hard cases, no doubt about that, but I had to admit I couldn't pinpoint any real differences between what those patients were doing and how I relied on my daily cups of coffee. It's just that coffee isn't illegal and doesn't cost $100 a day—though now Starbucks does make it easy to acquire quite an expensive habit!

Before long, I began to hate the labeling that went along with psychiatric medicine, when the names we attached to various collections of symptoms were so stigmatizing. It wasn't even medically necessary. The labels were descriptive, but not diagnostic. And as I've already said, no one had agreed on clear-cut solutions to the problems they described. So I resented my expected complicity in what amounted to high-level name-calling.

All of this brings me around to the second half of my mission with this book: reframing the standard psychiatric classifications into positive "types." I'm doing away with familiar curses like "anxiety," "clinical depression," and "obsession-compulsion" in favor of discussing the Stoic, Guardian, Warrior, Star, Dreamer, and Lover types. These archetypal names come from the positive aspects of various personality types. I choose to focus on many *positive* traits and tendencies we all have, leaving mainstream psychiatry to fixate on full-blown clinical presentations of the relatively rare negative aspects if they must. That also allows each of us to learn about ourselves and develop the best of our innate personalities while minimizing our weaknesses—all without having to wait for our behavior to swing to extremes.

How we talk about and think about anything affects how we experience the reality of it, so it is crucial to elevate the dialogue about brain chemistry out of the relentlessly negative terms we are all overexposed to. The change can be freeing in and of itself, but more important, it opens the door to understanding the full splendor of each and every type. Human nature is richly complex (thank goodness!), and these six categories encompass all of the wonder of human nature. Each person is predominantly one type. I don't want to oversimplify, so I want to make it clear that we all have dashes of other types, but you'll see one primary emphasis that goes a long way to encapsulating how you are and how you live your life.

If you care about your mental or emotional or psychological health—and the way it is intertwined with your physical state—most of what is already available to you accentuates the negative. It isn't a happy, well-balanced person, after all, who generally seeks out professional services. The Brain Chemistry Diet provides a happy, healthy alternative. Why not embrace the best in yourself and learn how to polish it up to shine as bright as possible?

Sure, when our brain chemistry is out of balance, there are pitfalls particular to each type that we have to watch out for. But that's just one little slice of the whole delicious pie. And we'll acknowledge that piece, of course. There's much to be learned there, for starters. But there are also ways to minimize the attendant vulnerabilities of any given type.

Before we go any further, I want to give you a brief overview of the brain:

The brain directs every voluntary activity in the body (motor functions and the musculoskeletal system), stimulates respiration, oversees digestion, manages growth and development, ensures tissue repair, and serves as Grand Central Station for the nervous system. (The brain contains 6 million nerve cells, fully half of the body's entire supply.) The brain is our interpreter of the outside world, monitoring information supplied by our five senses. It is also, of course, the center of our thoughts, feelings, and emotions. In fact, it is specially constructed for processing that complex mix.

The human brain is divided into two sections—a newer, outer layer called the neocortex or the cerebral cortex, and a more primitive interior region known as the Old Brain or archipallium. The neocortex, called "neo" because it is believed to have evolved more recently, is the seat of perception, learning, cognition, conscience, and morality. The Old Brain, including the hippocampus and brain stem, is where our moods and emotions dominate—fear, anxiety, happiness, love, excitement, and so on. All mammals have the equivalent of our Old Brain, but the large, overdeveloped, multi-wrinkled outside (the neocortex) sets humans apart.

Specialized nerve cells called neurons are the fundamental structure of the brain. The human brain has 100 billion neurons, and each one has as many as 100,000 links to other neurons. It transmits billions of messages between neurons every second. To get over the gap, or synapse, between neurons, those messages rely on chemicals known as neurotransmitters.

Neurons store neurotransmitters, releasing them in response to electrical signals. The neurotransmitter then attaches to receptors on nearby neurons, triggering another electrical signal. This is the way moods, thoughts, emotions, and impulses move throughout the brain.

Receptors on neurons are specific to certain neurotransmitters—like a lock and key. Only the correct neurotransmitter can make a match at any

The "Older" Brain

You never get any more neurons than you are born with. In fact, the brain loses nerve cells as it ages (and in the event of brain injury). Aging also cuts down on the number of extensions from the neurons (dendrites) that connect to other neurons, so communication between brain cells gets more difficult the older you get. Levels of some of the neurotransmitters charged with carrying positive feelings decrease. In addition, by age forty-five, levels of a powerful enzyme that is responsible for breaking down several types of neurotransmitters increase. The stepped-up breakdown can throw your brain chemistry out of balance and lead to, among many other things, a decrease in the general level of brain activity, interference with the ability to think and remember, and depression.

Certainly, none of this has to mean senility or the loss of mental function that we (wrongly) associate with getting older. You have plenty of neurons to keep you mentally strong for your entire life if you care for them well; and providing the materials for all the neurotransmitters you need is within your control. But aging can mean that your brain chemistry tips out of balance more easily if you don't provide proper nutrition. Looking at it another way, people may get away with sloppy eating habits in their youth, but those habits eventually catch up with them.

given receptor, and the correct pairing is required for the message to get through. Once it completes its mission, a neurotransmitter may be dissolved and discarded from the body or absorbed back into the neuron—or it may simply stay in circulation.

Virtually all neurons in the central nervous system, including the brain, are activated by excitatory neurotransmitters (glutamate being the most prevalent) and deactivated by inhibitory neurotransmitters, including gamma-aminobutyric acid (GABA) and glycine. The bulk of the highly organized information flow throughout the brain is regulated by nerve fibers containing the excitatory neurotransmitter glutamate ("glutamergic fibers") throughout the cerebral cortex. Other neurotransmitter pathways serve primarily to modulate the glutamate reactions.

While there's only one way for the message to get through—via a neurotransmitter between neurons—there are a host of ways for the message *not* to get through:

- There is not enough of the neurotransmitter, signals within the neuron will be unable to release it—or enough of it to do the job—into the synapse.
- Neurons are oversensitive and release too much of the neurotransmitter, swamping the system and not having enough for next time.
- Poor reabsorption of the neurotransmitter after it has delivered a message, so it isn't available to respond to the next signal.
- Too much of the neurotransmitter is broken down, so the message can't be completed, or there are no "leftovers" for the next message.
- The receptor is blocked by another molecule; therefore, the neurotransmitter cannot connect.
- The receiving neuron does not make the right receptor, or enough receptors, and the neurotransmitter (even the correct one in correct amounts) cannot deliver a message.

The disproportionate opportunities for failure, rather than success, make it that much more crucial that our brains get a constant supply of the correct neurotransmitters, and the raw materials for making them, in order to keep working smoothly. By and large, neurotransmitters become inactive once they're delivered a message, and they need to be replenished. Though they exist throughout the body, they cannot move into the brain from outside it, in order to protect it from fluctuations of neurotransmitters in the blood. Instead, they are made "on site"—in the brain, where and when they are needed. (It is also possible to have too much of a particular neurotransmitter, and breakdown is an important step in controlling this. Your body will make only what it needs from available materials.)

Neurotransmitters are made from amino acids (the building blocks of all proteins), which we get from the food we eat. Poor diet, then, can leave us without the ability to make the chemical messengers necessary for healthy brain function. Optimal nutrition, through high-quality food and, as necessary, supplements, maintains balance in the brain, which allows for a plentiful supply of the appropriate neurotransmitters and a general mood of well-being and comfort.

I've got many filing cabinets in my office—and garage—stuffed full of more than thirty years' worth of files on patients like Sarah. The details of each story are different, of course, and some are more dire than others. A few patients stay in therapy for months or even years, and many use prescription drugs of one kind or another to help handle their moods, but most find success with just a few visits and straightforward nutritional treatments.

Over the years, I've honed my recommendations into the individualized plans you now see presented in The Brain Chemistry Diet. These treatment strategies, designed to fit particular common biochemical scenarios, enable you to implement a comprehensive program of natural medicine that addresses specific psychological issues. At the same time, they allow you to escape the common trap of viewing our psychological states "through a glass, darkly," as if they are strictly pathological. This point of view brings only stress and stigmatization, so here we re-frame our mental states to reflect strengths as well as vulnerabilities.

Natural approaches to gently rebalance brain biochemistry can help us function optimally without sacrificing essential parts of ourselves on the

The Mind/Body Connection

Your brain physically changes in response to your experiences. Neurons develop new connections thanks to new sensations and even thoughts. While you learn something, or try something new, or go through something for the first time, your brain actually grows or alters its structure to accommodate that information.

altar of emotional well-being. One of the drawbacks of conventional psychopharmacology is that it may reduce symptoms at the expense of passion and creative fire, as Peter Kramer so eloquently explored in *Listening to Prozac*. Prozac in essence works *too* well, smothering all extremes of emotions and making you more brittle. But we need our emotions, including negative emotions, to survive—and evolve.

Furthermore, some symptoms we think are from mental illness are really from the drugs used to treat them (as with Sarah's fogginess). And too often we confuse addressing symptoms with treating the actual condition. Temporary relief is far from a cure.

I've treated thousands of patients suffering from psychiatric emotional difficulties over the last three decades with a comprehensive program of nutrition and natural medicine. In my clinical practice I've uncovered certain dietary practices and supplements that promote psychological health for people with a vast array of conditions. This book identifies six positive primary psychological types that require individualized dietary strategies, supplements, and lifestyle changes to achieve optimal wellness.

There's a chapter devoted to each of the types, containing descriptive profiles with delineation of both psychological strengths and psychiatric vulnerabilities. Real case histories from my files and analyses of historical and cultural figures who exemplify the type show the interconnectedness of the positive and negative, and help readers to identify themselves in a positive light.

An explanation of common imbalances in specific chemical systems in the brain typically associated with each type—and the markers that simple lab tests can look for to identify them—gives the biological underpinning of each type.

Each chapter also provides tailored dietary guidelines, including macronutrients like protein and carbohydrates, and specific foods that can rectify brain chemistry imbalances. The diets work in synergy with natural medicine solutions, including vitamins and minerals, amino acids, enzymes, fatty acids, and herbal remedies, all of which are detailed in the appropriate sections.

Psychological and spiritual practices, including particular schools of therapy and meditation, as well as other lifestyle changes that help each brain chemistry type to optimize strengths and minimize dysfunction, are also described.

Keep in mind that you'll no doubt see some of yourself in each profile, but you should follow the recommendations for your predominant type at any given time. No matter what your type, or how balanced or imbalanced you are right now, The Brain Chemistry Diet can bring you to optimal wellness.

Descartes was wrong in declaring, "I think, therefore I am." Really, there is no separate thinking from being. Popeye was closer to the truth: "I yam what I yam." Mind and body aren't parallel; they are one unit. We exist on several different planes at once. We are indivisibly thinking, being, and feeling at the same time. We have to divide up our world in order to make sense out of it, but we must not divide it so much that we forget about the wholeness of it all. The Brain Chemistry Diet serves as a reminder that what happens in the physical brain is what *is* the metaphysical "mind." It is our emotions, our thoughts, our mental states. Call it soul. Call it self. Call it you.

2

What Is Your Brain Type?

Before we go any further, you should find out what type you are, so you can get the most out of this book. The following statements help define your predominant character profile. Just circle the number of each one that is generally true of you. There are no right or wrong answers—only honest ones. The scoring key appears at the end. Don't peek!

(Note: While a sincere effort has been made for these statements to provide an accurate assessment, they have not been validated through scientific study and should be considered as providing only general guidelines.)

1. Everyone knows they can count on me.
2. I can't say "no."
3. When I am sad or angry, most times other people don't know it.
4. I don't need much in the way of material things.
5. I am good in a crisis.
6. I am not one to complain.
7. I am very considerate, always thinking of others' needs, often before my own.
8. I am pretty even-keeled—I don't get all worked up over things (good or bad).

9. When I do get upset, I tend to feel depressed.
10. I avoid conflict at all costs.
11. I am safety-conscious.
12. I like my life organized around a regular routine.
13. I know what is right and what is wrong; I live by my principles.
14. My friends say that I'm a worry wart.
15. I think over every option carefully before making a decision.
16. I am very careful with my money.
17. I am a collector.
18. I am very neat.
19. I am definitely not a quitter.
20. I put a premium on intelligence.
21. I like to be spontaneous.
22. I am a risk taker.
23. I can be very persuasive.
24. Feeling good and having a good time are high on my list of priorities.
25. I have a hot temper.
26. I always do the right thing.
27. I am more a *doer* than a thinker or a talker.
28. When I get upset, I usually get angry.
29. When I'm on a mission, I don't let anything get in my way.
30. I am decisive.
31. I am an optimist.
32. I can talk a blue streak.
33. I am very active; I've got a lot of energy.
34. I am fun to be around.
35. I like to be the center of attention.
36. If I get sad or angry, everyone around me is sure to know about it.
37. I am intuitive.
38. When my mood changes, it can do so pretty dramatically.

39. I like to have a leadership role in things.
40. I am intense and passionate.
41. I am shy.
42. I am good at what I do.
43. I have high moral standards.
44. I keep to myself.
45. Material things mean nothing to me.
46. My feelings are easily hurt.
47. I feel a lot of people just don't understand me.
48. I can't stand anger.
49. Spirituality is important to me.
50. I am more a thinker than a doer.
51. I am an outgoing person.
52. I like to live life to the fullest.
53. Sex is one of life's great pleasures.
54. I can be fickle.
55. I am "in touch with" my emotions.
56. I enjoy flirting.
57. When I get upset, I tend to feel anxious.
58. Other people tend to be drawn to me.
59. I am a "people person"; one of those "people who need people."
60. I would do anything for love.

What is more important here is the pattern of your answers. If you look back, the numbers you have circled are probably roughly clustered together. Here's what those clusters mean:

If you have circled six or more of statements 1–10, you are a Stoic.
If you have circled six or more of statements 11–20, you are a
    Guardian.
If you have circled six or more of statements 21–30, you are a
    Warrior.
If you have circled six or more of statements 31–40, you are a Star.

If you have circled six or more of statements 41–50, you are a Dreamer.

If you have circled six or more of statements 51–60, you are a Lover.

You may have more than one cluster—which is normal, since we all have parts of all types within us. Your dominant type is the group with the most items circled. In the unlikely event that you have more than one group with six "true" answers, your dominant character will be the one with the highest number circled. If there's a tie for the most "true"s, even if under six, you have more than one dominant type.

To help you understand how all the types fit together, it helps to think of them as forming a wheel:

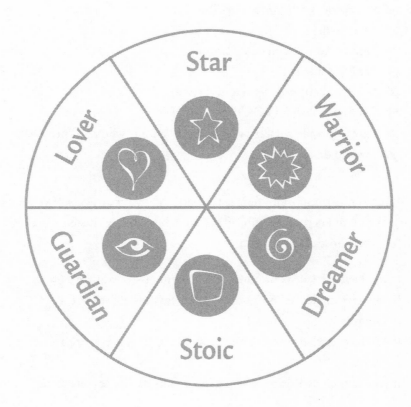

The types on one half of the wheel—Lover-Star-Warrior—are outer-directed, or extroverted, while the other half—Guardian-Stoic-Dreamer—contains more inner-directed types. Your "runner-up" type is probably in the same hemisphere as your dominant type. Your smaller cluster (or clusters)—your secondary type(s)—most likely falls immediately next to your dominant type and is extremely unlikely to fall directly opposite it.

The Six Character Profiles

All humans have the same basic brain structure and function. But if we look more closely at the outward expression of brain function, we can identify the six distinct character profiles mentioned above. The following chapters are devoted to one character profile each, and explore in detail the advantages and weak points of each. In this chapter, I'd just like to give you a brief overview of each profile to give you the lay of the land, in general, and help point you toward the chapter you'll be most interested in.

We all have aspects of each type at least at some time, but you'll find that one type predominates most of the time. You should follow, then, the recommendations for your predominant type, within the framework of a generally healthy diet, as discussed above. But you'll be able to learn something from each type that you can apply as it comes up for you, even as you focus on your main category. So I want to stress the importance of reading about all the types—you'll glean something from each.

In the brief descriptions here, and in the chapters that follow, I'll be showing you both the type "in balance" and the type "in trouble." Your type tells you a lot about how you are in the world, your approach to life, where you draw strength, and how you face problems. As long as your brain chemistry stays in balance, any type can serve you well. But your type also predicts where and how you'll run into trouble if your brain chemistry gets out of whack. Just as each type has distinct positive traits associated with it, each also has a characteristic way of breaking down under stress (i.e., imbalanced biochemistry). So keep in mind that it would be a mistake to say, for example, that a Star has manic-depressive qualities. But a Star *in trouble* would indeed be diagnosed as having bipolar disorder—or, in milder versions, a tendency toward bipolar behaviors.

But it is also worth noting that, whatever the symptoms, the negative expressions of each type all trace back to depression, anxiety, and anger. No matter what they look like, specifically, we all have the same handful of core problems. We just react to them differently. The mechanism is the same, but the weak points are different. The same things set off different types, but then they go off in different ways.

So, before we really dig in, here's an overview of the six types.

THE STOIC

Stoics are by far the most common type. Not that it's a scientific sampling, but I'd guess that about half the people I see in my office are Stoics. More women are Stoics than men.

The phrase that always comes to my mind when I'm talking about Stoics is "salt of the earth." These are the kind of people who hold everything together. They soldier through any difficulty. They get the job done. They don't complain. They don't say "No." They are attentive to detail and are usually quite organized. They think of others first. After a dinner party, when the other guests are taking their ease, the Stoic is in the kitchen, quietly loading the dishwasher (without having been asked). When you're really up against it with a project at the office, the person you lean on for last-minute, exactingly professional work over the weekend is (I'm betting) a Stoic.

When Stoics' brain chemistry tips out of balance, they are subject to chronic depression. Since Stoics don't cry until the pain is pretty intense (they are stoical, after all), when they run into trouble it is often quite severe. Problems often come up when they've given too much to others and haven't considered themselves anywhere in the equation. Sometimes you have to think of yourself first, and learning to do that can help Stoics right themselves. But more commonly, malnutrition of one sort or another is what sends them over the edge. Either way, balancing brain chemistry through nutritional therapy is in order. (This will be a recurring theme with each type, so you may as well get used to it!) It can also help keep your brain chemistry functioning optimally so you don't find yourself drifting to the negative extremes of your type, whatever it may be.

THE GUARDIAN

Like the Stoic, the Guardian is other-directed. Guardians have a healthy concern for others, focused on their own safety and well-being as well as that of their loved ones. They are effective manipulators of the business of life. Again like Stoics, they are attentive to detail. They are forever watchful, on guard for dangers from without or within. Guardians have retirement accounts, insurance policies, and a basement stash of bottled water and extra batteries. They are the type of people who test the smoke alarm four times a year, without fail.

Usually, all this makes Guardians steady, reliable, and secure. But when their brain chemistry gets disordered, their tendency toward constant vigilance leaves them vulnerable to chronic anxiety or depression that expresses itself as obsession/compulsion. Obsession/compulsion is really a kind of defense against depression or anxiety, and a Guardian won't really feel anxiety or depression until that defense breaks down. In trouble, Guardians can lose perspective on usually intelligent, sensible rituals, like hand washing, or tuning off lights, or making lists (a favorite activity of Guardians), and perform them disproportionately, spending so much time on these obsessive rituals that they get less and less productive work done.

Imbalance of neurotransmitters can exaggerate natural character traits. When that happens, Guardians become bogged down in a thousand contingencies and can get totally paralyzed by ambivalence, deeply mired in considering every option. They worry endlessly about what else they can do or what they may have left undone. A Guardian in trouble doesn't have the ability to realize that someone else will take care of some problems, or that some things can't be foreseen or forestalled. They never acknowledge, "This is bigger than me." They carry the weight of the world on their shoulders.

THE WARRIOR

Where Guardians and Stoics focus their concern on others—though their basic goal is to preserve their own situation—Warriors are ready to risk everything in pursuit of a cause. And Warriors are usually dedicated to some mission and will do whatever it takes to make it a success. Everybody has a friend who is the Warrior type. Warriors tend to be pleasant, "up" people to be around—fun-loving and charming. They are very persuasive and passionate about their beliefs. They tend not to have a heavy critical sense about themselves and don't waste any time thinking about behaving "correctly."

Guardians and Stoics live well-ordered lives, but Warriors are creatures of impulse and tend toward extremes. They go to Vegas for a few days at the drop of a hat, or bring their lovers big bouquets when it isn't a birthday or anniversary, or stay up all night engrossed in an argument. A Warrior does what he feels like (and Warriors are more often men than women).

Warriors are often in the military, or religious leaders, or political crusaders, or salespeople, or entrepreneurs, or CEOs. Whatever the field, for Warriors it is never a nine-to-five gig, but a twenty-four-hour-a-day game. The mission isn't always about duty (that's more the domain of the Stoic), and it isn't always deadly serious. Whatever it is, it is something they get very excited about. Warriors can be the ones up in the bleachers at every single home game, with their bodies painted in team colors, and the fight song on their home answering machines. Or Warriors can be stage parents bent on seeing their little ones in starring roles.

A Warrior with out-of-balance brain chemistry runs the risk of undesirable behavior. When their neurotransmitters go awry, what is usually spontaneous and delightful slides downhill into explosive anger, animal desires, and even violence. We all have impulses of rage sometimes, but Warriors in trouble are less likely to check it. They go after whatever they can get, fair means or foul. They'll con you if they can—and kill you if they can't (metaphorically and, on occasion, literally). Not only will they do socially unacceptable things, they'll brag about them afterward. When they are in balance, they may harness the positive power of anger for a righteous cause, but out of balance, their rage may not be "for cause" and is surely poorly controlled. Warriors in trouble are bullies and operate with the Machiavellian attitude that the end justifies the means (whatever the means, and no matter the desired end).

Serious psychopaths are Warriors in the deepest kind of trouble, but you know the more familiar signs of a Warrior in breakdown mode too: the person cutting in line at the bank (*I'm late enough as it is!*), the sales clerk who steals clothes from the shop (*They couldn't run this place without me, and they pay me peanuts—I deserve it!*), the person taking the last serving from the dish before it's been passed all the way around the table (*I'm hungry!*), the person set off by a near-miss fender bender (*What are you trying to do, kill me?*). The Stoic worries too much about what others think—but the Warrior doesn't worry enough.

THE STAR

Stars are the movers and shakers of our world. Relatively rare in number, they tend to be the bosses, the team captains, the generals, the larger-than-life celebrities—the leaders, capable of rallying others to higher goals. The "everyday" Star might be the operator who engages you while she looks up the number you requested, or the "fun dictator" in your group of friends, or the dearly loved, astoundingly peppy coach of your daughter's hapless soccer team. They are optimistic, showing amazing fortitude when others have given up hope. They have a tremendous ability to love—including loving themselves greatly—and love deeply, and they have an overwhelming concern for everyone. Stars are passionate. They are intense, active, and energizing to be around. They make your life more exciting.

When all is working well, Stars embody the intuition, drive, and instinct of the "primitive" brain in happy combination with the logic and thinking of the "new" brain. This fusion of emotion and reason modulates both, and mixes them in a beautiful panoply. That's what allows Stars to create something out of nothing—a new industry, a work of art, a unique process. Stars are not only great creators but also great workers (unlike Dreamers). They get things done in this world. They make things happen. Like a Warrior, a Star is fun-loving and can get wrapped up in a goal.

The Star in trouble becomes depressed, with a component of mania that is really a defense against the depression. When out-of-balance brain chemistry creates this bipolar depression, the Star's usually appealing attributes are exaggerated enough to become unpleasant. In a manic extreme, a Star in trouble may be dominating, obnoxious, shrill, and exhausting. They can totally wear you out with their overwhelming outbursts of energy. They can talk for hours on a topic that might normally sustain a five-minute conversation. The true danger in a manic phase is lack of judgment, and an out-of-control Star may do things that aren't sensible—like spending a fortune in a scheme to beat the tables in Atlantic City or repainting the house without consulting the other occupants.

At the other extreme, a Star's depression looks quite different from a Stoic's. A Stoic gets quietly depressed, and it can be difficult to tell they are even depressed by the way they behave—it may be that only lab tests will reveal how out of balance they are. They can even have a "smiling depression"—culturally, they want to be nice and pleasant, even when they are discussing the depths of their despair (if you can get them to do that at all). But not the Star. It is never hard to believe that a Star is depressed. For Stars, their depression is a big, dramatic thing. When they are in balance, Stars will complain when they are down, and that freedom of expression is usually a good thing—it can clear the air or lead you to getting whatever help you need. But when Stars are out of balance, they can talk of nothing else and insist on drawing anyone within earshot into the storm.

THE DREAMER

The Dreamer is the rarest of types, even less common than the Star. The greatest visionaries of our society are Dreamers. They dream big dreams no one else would even conceive of. They have sharp brains and a highly developed moral sense. Still, Dreamers are humble. They are generally noncompetitive and don't have much use for material things (aside from whatever is necessary to fulfill their vision). Dreamers are terribly concerned with everybody else's welfare. They are egoless and easily influenced by their surroundings. They are exquisitely sensitive, and easily slighted, even when no harm was intended. In general, Dreamers are nice to be around—pleasant, sweet, and gentle. But they are not highly social, and often find spending too much time around others to be overstimulating. They are introspective and well suited to solitude.

Not all Dreamers are in the change-the-world line of work. They may have any kind of job and usually will perform quite responsibly, but really do it just to pay the rent—and all the while, they are basically up there living in their heads. Dreamers are good at jobs others might find lonely, such as something that requires sitting in front of a computer screen all day or working in a remote area. Dreamers give away money even if they don't have much to begin with. They pass up a piece of cake if they fear there won't be enough to go around. They believe the best about everyone and want the best for them. Dreamers are meditators, whether or not they follow any formal practice.

When Dreamers have out-of-balance brain chemistry, they tend toward borderline personality disorder and, in the most extreme cases, schizophrenia. They can get completely absorbed in their internal world. They may become alienated and prideful, and suffer from loneliness. They know they are different from everybody else—smarter, better—but feel that their greatness is unrecognized. They can neglect themselves, going for days without eating or bathing.

Dreamers in trouble are easily angered. Anger is a common problem for most types in trouble. The angry Stoic recognizes anger and suppresses it into depression, for example. Or the Warrior knows what to do with anger, yelling or punching, releasing emotion for better or worse. When Dreamers are angry, it is usually out of self-defense. They may not even know they are angry or may try to rise above anger by creating a whole different reality in their minds. To an even greater extent than Stoics, they avoid confrontation at all costs. As a result, they can't deal with small matters directly, and those small things then tend to fester until they explode. In the extreme, running away from anger, Dreamers in trouble move into a dreamworld, avoiding unpleasant reality by creating their own.

THE LOVER

The Lover is every bit as outgoing and people-oriented as the Dreamer is introspective and cerebral. Lovers really like and enjoy people, and others usually find Lovers very attractive. Lovers are emphatic and, well, loving. They are aware of and comfortable with their sexuality, and have been known to use it to get what they want. They'd do anything to avoid hurting the feelings of those they care about. They are flirtatious, warm, friendly, approachable, and exciting to be around. More women are Lovers than men, though of course there are plenty of male Lovers.

Lovers can relate their love in a warm, personal way, whether one-on-one or even in front of large groups. That's why movie stars are often Lovers. (Though they also make great teachers, social workers, nurses, and so on—and earn great tips when they wait tables and high commissions when they are in sales.) We all love to watch Lovers. They make us feel loved.

Lovers generally do not get depressed over the long haul, because they react right away to injury. They are emotionally expressive. They let their feelings out, and get and give immediate feedback. But when their brain chemistry is out of balance, Lovers can cripple themselves with exaggerated reactions, and they are prone to anxiety, panic attacks, and hysterical behavior. They may have physical symptoms not traceable to any physiological condition and, in extreme cases, may even undergo complicated or painful (but usually unnecessary) medical treatments in pursuit of relief. They can become overly dependent on other people, and other people's actions and attitudes, and any small negative hits them like a ton of bricks. Lovers in trouble can't handle anger and somatize it. They feel jumpy, queasy, or get rapid heartbeats or "butterflies" in their stomachs. A Lover in trouble tends to be passive-aggressive. As if following Shakespeare's dictum, "All's fair in love and war," Lovers in trouble can be deceptive, sometimes lying and cheating to gain their passion.

Armed with this most basic knowledge of your own personal type, you are ready for the full chapter of strategies for maximizing your potential—the nutritional strategies that support you in optimal overall health, keeping the Dreamers dreaming big dreams, the Stars shining bright, the Warriors at fighting weight, and so on. You'll learn how to eat, the daily supplements to take to be all you can be and to smooth over the inevitable rough spots and make them fewer and farther between (and easier to cope with when they do occur), the interventions you can press into service if you slip out of balance and into trouble, and the lifestyle changes that can also help you bring out your best.

The idea is to make the most of your innate tendencies, ensuring a stable balance in your brain chemistry—and your personality—and to maximize all that is best in you and protect any weaknesses. I believe in gently re-balancing brain chemistry *naturally* rather than attempting to get rid of symptoms with pharmaceutical cures that are sometimes worse than the disorders they are aimed at—and offer nothing in the way of prevention or self-improvement. Even for the majority of people, who don't reach the ex-tremes but have to contend with the plusses and minuses of their own brain chemistry, staying in balance is the key.

To help you extract all that from this book, I have a few recommendations:

1. First, identify your type, through the self-assessment and by reading the initial descriptions.

2. Read all of the chapters in order (you learn from every type), then go back and read about your dominant type again to really absorb it. You will glean a lot from your secondary types—and also from your opposite. It will benefit you to be aware of your weaknesses as well as your strengths. And the more you understand the types of the people around you, the better. Keep the image of the wheel in your mind as you proceed to chapters other than the one for your pri-mary type, and use it to get a perspective on how what you are read-ing relates to you.

3. If you are not a Stoic, refer to the Stoic chapter for more details on the supplements and interventions for all types. Because the Stoic is the most common type, that chapter comes first in the book and contains the most detailed information about most supplements and interventions. So it will be useful regardless of your type.

4. In some cases, you'll need to refer to some other chapters for more details (to limit repetition of the same background information in

different chapters). Where that is the case, I've pointed you in the right direction in the text.

5. Keep in mind, as you are reading about the specific cases I discuss, that although you may be struck by the extremes of behavior I see in so many patients, for the most part, these are actually the milder variations I've dealt with. The people most likely to seek professional help are those in the deepest trouble. What I want you to notice, though, is how the natural remedies work even in these, the toughest cases. Their power is just the greater in more garden-variety imbalances, and better still when pressed into service before real problems strike. That's their finest usage: keeping brain chemistry in balance, playing to your strengths.

6. Although each chapter describes the "Brain Chemistry Markers" for the type with specifics on how to interpret lab results, you only need to get this sort of workup if you have tipped out of balance and into trouble and/or if you need the information to help you determine which intervention may be best for you. If you are basically in balance and just looking to know how to support that balance nutritionally, you don't need to know these specific readings.

7. First, I want to emphasize that, when you are in trouble, you should be under the supervision of a medical professional still. Each chapter lists many possible interventions for the type in trouble. While it may be theoretically possible to use all of them together, I recommend taking only one intervention at a time. (The Daily Supplements are designed to be taken all together.) I'm including all of them just to help you understand the full range of your options. Just as with prescription drugs, it may take a little trial and error to find what works best for you. By considering your symptoms and by reading the descriptions of the interventions, you will learn what direction to go in. You may ultimately decide to combine two (or even more) interventions, but I don't recommend doing so until you are familiar with how your body reacts to each one separately. And if you do combine, keep in mind that most interventions will act syn-

ergistically, so you'll need smaller doses of any given one than you would if you were using that one alone.

8. Remember that most of my patients—and all of the patients in any of the research I cite—are "in trouble." That is why they are patients. But the benefit of this program is much broader than that. In fact, my hope is that most readers will use this book *before* they are in trouble, seeing it primarily not as treatment but as prevention. That's where the most power lies—staying in balance and, from there, accessing the very best of yourself. If it seems that you keep reading about negative examples or cases, please keep this in mind.

3

The
Stoic

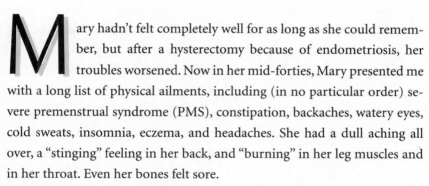

Mary hadn't felt completely well for as long as she could remember, but after a hysterectomy because of endometriosis, her troubles worsened. Now in her mid-forties, Mary presented me with a long list of physical ailments, including (in no particular order) severe premenstrual syndrome (PMS), constipation, backaches, watery eyes, cold sweats, insomnia, eczema, and headaches. She had a dull aching all over, a "stinging" feeling in her back, and "burning" in her leg muscles and in her throat. Even her bones felt sore.

It didn't come as much of a surprise when Mary wrapped up her spiel (well rehearsed from visiting many doctors) by saying she was depressed. With all those aches and pains, who wouldn't be? As she unfolded the rest of her story, I also was not surprised to learn that she fit the Stoic profile to a T. This chapter begins by laying out her case, and through it you'll learn much of what there is to know about Stoic biochemistry and balance. After that, I'll back up to the scientific details of Stoic brain chemistry markers, and then present dietary guidelines and supplement recommendations for Stoics so you can do for yourself what Mary did. Finally, we'll get to the mind/body strategies most suited to this type.

Typically, Mary devoted most of her energy to the well-being of others, to the point where she neglected her own. She got more done in a day than I do in a week, avoided conflict at all costs, and never thought of herself first. And she never complained. In fact, she rarely expressed emotion—at least not negative emotion.

Mary's husband was an extremely wealthy man and a real big shot in their town. She'd once been his secretary, and though she no longer worked with him, it often seemed a lot like he was still the boss and she the underling. He was famous for his temper tantrums, and she'd long since learned to listen to his occasional tirades and provide sympathy for the pressures that running the company put on him.

Mary kept things running smoothly on the home front, never mentioning her own problems to her husband. She kept an immaculate and fashionable home, entertained friends (and company clients) frequently, coordinated the multiple activities of her two school-aged children, and did all the household and personal financial paperwork (in her perfect handwriting). She had a wide circle of friends who knew they could always count on her. She was proud of being prompt, detail oriented, and organized.

She didn't include it in her description of herself, but it was clear that Mary was the kind of woman you'd call "sweet": soft-spoken, calm, friendly, and dependable. And she wasn't one to call attention to herself. Even in grade school, she had never raised her hand, though she kept bringing home A's on her report cards. Her parents never had to "shush" her or tell her to settle down the way they scolded her brother. She never had angry outbursts like her husband, though she noticed how it seemed to help him get everything out of his system. And she never burst into tears like some of her friends. She told me everyone always said she was very even keeled.

Though the town Mary and her family lived in wasn't large, Mary was prominent in local "society." She had all the trappings that came with that role—membership at an exclusive country club, regular mentions in the local paper, expensive clothes, a high-end car, and elite private school memberships for her two kids. Some of that she enjoyed, and some she just endured. "I'm really just a simple country girl," she told me. She put on a good show but didn't feel quite at home in this high-profile life.

Athletics was Mary's only outlet, and she was an avid jogger and tennis player—or had been, until the pain got to be too much. It struck me that she had been literally running away from her life, and when she lost the ability to do that, her depression really sank in.

Abandoning her usual level of activity also meant that Mary was gaining unwanted weight and was up to twenty pounds more than her usual set point. She'd never done anything in particular to control her weight, and the exercise she enjoyed had always kept her slim. Now she didn't know what to do to stop, and reverse, the weight gain. Besides that, she said she was always hungry.

Mary told me that she had a pretty healthy diet—she'd been watching her cholesterol and fat since the days when oat bran became fashionable, mostly avoided red meat and eggs, and worried about the constantly changing butter-vs.-margarine recommendations. While none of that caution was wrong, per se, her diet was now heavy on pasta, breads, fat-free yogurt, and frozen yogurt. Pretzels seemed to be a staple (fat free!). You wouldn't catch much in the way of meat or dairy fat crossing Mary's lips, but what she ate was loaded with white flour and white sugar.

Even though Mary's diet was healthier in some ways than the diets of most Americans (she never heard the words, "Would you like an order of fries with that?"), what she was eating was giving her chronic malnutrition. When she removed natural fats from her diet, she also removed the fat-soluble vitamins (A, D, E, and K). Those vitamins are coenzymes that make the body's metabolic machinery run, and without enough of them, the metabolism slows. In short, Mary's diet was making her overweight, sluggish, and fatigued. These vitamins are no less important in the brain, and their lack, combined with the excess of sugars she was getting, was tipping her brain chemistry out of balance. As is typical of Stoics, that made her subject to depression.

Mary's struggle with depression had been lifelong. Some days were better than others. When her depression got worse, her physical symptoms usually worsened as well, especially the PMS. Most of her assorted aches and pains came with age, she felt, but her menstrual difficulties were a long-standing foe. Mary thought she probably began menopause in her late thirties and wondered if she wasn't still going through it (the hysterectomy left her with one ovary).

Know Your Type

I did a complete series of lab tests on Mary, and while I waited for the lab results (before I prescribed anything), I talked with her a bit about the Stoic personality. She was already familiar with the downside—suppressed emotions, ever-increasing demands from others, depression—but I wanted her to see the positive aspects she embodied as well.

Extreme capability is one hallmark of a Stoic, and Mary had that in spades. It got her into trouble sometimes—taking on more than she truly could handle, or feeling guilty that she couldn't handle something—but on the whole it had served her well. She was good in a crisis—another Stoic trait. No matter what hardship came her way, she always found a way to soldier on—just like a Stoic. She was very giving and extremely supportive.

Like all Stoics, Mary was other-oriented and had a finely tuned sense of duty. The danger there is neglecting yourself, a trap Mary had walked right into. Stoics don't spend money on themselves, and when they do, it's rarely on vanities or luxuries. They don't want to call and bother you, no matter what it is they actually need, or how reasonable the request, or how close a friend you are. They drive themselves to the airport. They feed their pets before they eat. They ask others to do something only when the favor is in the service of a higher calling.

Many Stoics are nine-to-five types. Most aren't concerned with worldly goods, though some do quite well financially. They take care of the nuts-and-bolts business of work. They make the world go round.

With my patients who are thoughtful and open to talk therapy, I like to provide a full picture—plusses and minuses—of their type, whatever it may be. I do this only briefly and let the information "sit" with them to use if it seems to fit. Though I am a psychiatrist, I do very little in the way of extended talk therapy. In most cases, nutritional counseling, requiring maybe three visits, is all my patients need to rebalance their own brain chemistry. Improved brain chemistry creates a more positive, serene mental state. Only a few also choose to pursue talking.

Almost everyone seems to welcome a chance to broaden their own ideas of themselves. By the time they are in my office, most people are very stuck in the negative corners of their personalities—it's what motivates them to seek help. Restoring a well-rounded vision of their innate tendencies is usually one piece of the healing process. It only takes a brief conversation to plant that seed, though it is then up to the individual to nurture it to the point where it bears fruit.

NUTRITIONAL DEFICIENCIES

In Mary's case, after our initial discussion of the positive aspects of the Stoic personality, our focus remained on nutritional solutions. The quickest test I do with any patient, and the first thing I did with Mary, is to look at the tongue. The appearance of the tongue gives a surprising amount of information. Mary's tongue was somewhere between purple and magenta, a shade that often indicates a shortage of riboflavin. It showed slight cracking, meaning she needed the B-complex vitamins in general, and niacin in particular. A shortage of B vitamins, including thiamine (B1), riboflavin (B2), niacin (B3), pantothenic acid (B5), pyridoxine (B6), folic acid, and cobalamin (B12), is often involved in depression and fatigue.

Mary's tongue was clean of mucus, so I wasn't too worried about food allergies or candidiasis (yeast infection), which I might otherwise have suspected. In fact, a blood test for candida came up negative. Blood tests for food allergies came back positive for wheat, and mildly positive for chicken, codfish, coffee, and baker's (but not brewer's) yeast. Although the allergies were not severe, I recommended Mary avoid, or at least cut back on, these foods. With the exception of the fish, these were items she relied on heavily.

I also did tests for chronic fatigue syndrome and fibromyalgia, including checking for Epstein-Barr Virus and Herpes I and II. I did a complete vitamin panel, too. The results of that blood test put all the nutrients within "normal" ranges, so she had no dire deficiencies. But keeping in mind that "normal" is not at all the same as "optimal," and remembering my physical exam of the tongue showing evidence of chronic vitamin deficiency, I recommended that she take a B-complex supplement to ensure that she got enough thiamine (vitamin B1), niacin (vitamin B3), and riboflavin (vitamin B2).

Thiamine deficiency can cause stinging or burning sensations or general soreness to the touch, much like what Mary was experiencing, so despite "normal" levels, I thought her body might not be getting as much as it needed. A lack of riboflavin can cause watering eyes, so again I was skeptical that Mary was getting enough through her diet. I prescribed niacin because it boosts serotonin levels, the same as prescription antidepressants are supposed to do. (In fact, niacin indirectly makes new serotonin, while drugs like Prozac and Paxil are selective serotonin reuptake inhibitors, meaning they just prevent the destruction of some of the serotonin already in the body—they can't make additional serotonin.) The B-complex vitamins are also good general stress busters. Vitamin C is, too, and is also good for pain relief, so I suggested she take that as well.

Mary was not a smoker and never had been. She did drink some alcohol, about one beer or one glass of wine a week, she guessed. Alcohol can deplete minerals, though probably not at the level Mary was consuming. People notoriously underestimate the amount of alcohol they consume, however, particularly women, so I did suggest to Mary that she might want to more strictly limit the amount she drank.

Mary's serotonin levels were at the low end of normal. Cortisol is typically high in Stoics, as is histamine, another neurotransmitter. Although Mary came to see me as if she were just coming for a general physical checkup, it eventually became clear that overcoming depression was really at the top of her agenda. She was a covert depressive. You wouldn't have known she was depressed from having a general conversation with her. She didn't "act depressed." In fact, she was usually smiling. That's often true of a Stoic, and serotonin levels on the low end, but not dramatically dropped, fit right in with that. Even Stoics with rock-bottom levels of serotonin might show up in my office *looking* happy, and more moderate serotonin levels make that even more likely.

Blood tests showed that Mary's magnesium level was at the low end of normal (which, again, has nothing to do with what is optimal anyway). Magnesium deficiency can result in depression and irritability. Hair analysis revealed that Mary had low levels of zinc—and generally low levels of minerals—but high levels of copper. The range of normal for both zinc and copper is very wide, but the most important numbers to keep in mind are the ratio between the two, which should ideally be close to 1:1, with just a bit more zinc than copper. For most doctors, Mary's copper levels wouldn't have rung any alarm bells, since it was in the normal range—the high end of normal, but still normal. But blood tests confirmed an imbalance in the zinc-to-copper ratio—nearly twice as much copper as zinc—and because the body does all it can to keep the blood normal at all costs (homeostasis), any abnormality in the blood shows a glaring problem.

Copper is a stimulant, and the right amount helps our brains to be sharp and smart. But excessively high levels can result in an overexcited, over-stimulated mind and, as a consequence, nervous exhaustion. Having the copper-to-zinc ratio out of whack toxically affects even someone with a normal blood copper level, causing "racing mind" insomnia, agitated depression, and even paranoia and psychotic states. A high copper level is typical in chronic depression—and of Stoics—and is far more common than having too much zinc.

Anything that stresses you raises your copper and lowers your zinc levels. Tea, coffee, and chocolate all raise copper levels (probably because of the effects of caffeine, which are pretty much the same as stress). Coffee itself is a good source of copper, and in Mary's case, I suspected it was a major culprit. She had a three-cup-a-day coffee habit and told me she liked her coffee strong! I recommended zinc supplements to gain sufficient levels and, even more important, to restore the balance with copper.

HYPOGLYCEMIA

I also ordered a five-hour glucose tolerance test for Mary. Sixty to 70 percent of the patients I see are hypoglycemic, thanks to the typical American diet, so I often suspect it. Fatigue is also a common complaint in hypoglycemia, so Mary had to say no more for me to test her.

That test revealed that she had "flat curve" hypoglycemia, a pattern of low blood sugar characteristic of Stoics. While bipolar people (manic-depressives) with low blood sugar tend to have erratic fluctuations in blood sugar levels (which will be further discussed in Chapter 6: The Star), Stoics tend to have unrelentingly low levels. In healthy, non-hypoglycemic people, blood sugar levels go up by 50 percent or more in response to a large dose of sugar and then gradually return to normal. In standard hypoglycemia (reactive hypoglycemia), levels will rise in the same way but then fall much too low. In flat curve hypoglycemia, blood sugar levels don't rise much, if at all, even in response to eating sugar. Rather, they are low, and stay low.

Hypoglycemia—low blood sugar—is sometimes called hyperinsulinism because it results from an overworked pancreas. The pancreas makes insulin, which is necessary for processing sugar. In low blood sugar, the pancreas is actually working *too well* under the stress of large amounts of sugar—just like a person under work-related stress might initially rise to the challenge by working harder. Excessive insulin secretion sends the blood sugar suddenly low. In flat curve hypoglycemia, the pancreas is so primed and ready to handle any sugar coming its way that it responds quickly, and comes on like gangbusters, with enough insulin to handle a seven-course meal, even if all you've had was a couple of chocolates or a tall latte. Small snacks like that don't give you the continuing release of sugar into the blood that a long meal does, so your blood sugar goes up dramatically and then, because of the excessive outpouring of insulin, plummets dramatically.

Just like a person working too hard to get the job done, after enough abuse, the pancreas will burn out or break down, particularly if it doesn't get the nutrients it needs for optimal functioning (like the macronutrient protein; the micronutrients chromium, zinc, and other minerals; and thiamine [vitamin B1], pyridoxine [vitamin B6], and other vitamins). Then you have an even more severe problem: diabetes—high blood sugar because of inadequate insulin production. This is why hypoglycemia, left unchecked, may be a sign of even more serious problems to come.

With the hypoglycemic diet, the idea is to de-stress the pancreas—and stop overproduction of insulin—by giving it much less sugar to process. With more reasonable demands on it, the body re-regulates itself. In most cases, after an initial two to six months on a strict diet, you can loosen your controls somewhat without any problem. But first you have to break the destructive cycle.

Hypoglycemia is often a factor in brain chemistry imbalance in all the types, so the diets described for each one are suitable for handling hypoglycemia as long as you are diligent about controlling sugars and eating frequently.

Insomnia

Hypoglycemia can cause difficulty sleeping, which Mary was experiencing. When the blood sugar gets low, the adrenal glands release adrenaline, which brings stored sugar into the bloodstream, bringing the blood sugar to a normal level. In addition to regulating blood sugar, adrenaline, also known as epinephrine, causes an alarm reaction—and may therefore waken the restless sleeper. High copper contributes to similar problems, so balancing Mary's copper and zinc levels would help her as well. But the single most important thing for Mary's sleeping was a diet to correct her hypoglycemia.

To relieve her insomnia, I recommended she drink a cup of warm milk at bedtime. In addition to being a good source of protein and calming minerals like calcium, milk contains a natural sedative, tryptophan. Warm foods are better digested and absorbed than cold foods and are relaxing (as long as they are not so hot as to be stimulating). Finally, a cup of warm milk is simply a "comfort food" for many people, calming by pleasant association with hearth and home.

The key elements of a healthy diet for anyone with hypoglycemia are reducing refined carbohydrates, especially refined sugar, and increasing protein. In addition, eating frequently helps keep blood sugar levels on an even keel. I recommend 5 to 7 small meals a day, and a healthy protein-rich snack (like a slice of turkey or a glass of milk) at the first sign of a dip in mood, which probably indicates that you're also experiencing a dip in blood sugar.

Alcohol contributes to hypoglycemia, so limiting it, as Mary agreed to, will also help. Coffee and tea can act as mild antidepressants, but for Mary her coffee habit clearly had negative consequences that outweighed any potential benefits.

Malnutrition and hypoglycemia are related by association, not cause and effect. The malnutrition that causes hypoglycemia also causes depression. In severe depression, there may be under-eating and weight loss because of lack of appetite or interest. Other people try to cope with depression by overeating junk food. In either case, malnutrition results. Paying attention to hypoglycemia is one of the quickest ways out of depression, as correcting the malnutrition it heralds will solve both problems.

GETTING BETTER ALL THE TIME

On this diet, and taking the supplements I recommended, Mary started to feel better within a month. In addition to reducing refined carbohydrates in general, she also cut out all wheat because of her allergy. She stopped drinking alcohol altogether but couldn't seem to do away with coffee (though she agreed to make it weaker). Coffee can deplete thiamine, but taking a 500-mg supplement twice a day was enough for Mary to wipe out her deficiency, and the burning sensations went away. Her various aches and pains let up, which I attribute to her taking thiamine and vitamin C.

Mary gradually built up the amount of niacin she took, doubling the dosage each day for three days, beginning with 300 mg a day (100 mg with a meal, three times a day). She experienced the niacin flush—dilation of the small capillaries in the skin, which can feel like a hot flash and make you look as if you have a sunburn—but didn't find it as upsetting as some people do. In fact, she said she sort of enjoyed the "rush" of it, so she didn't need one of the "flushless" forms. Since she was having no side effects (some people can't tolerate higher doses, and experience nausea, diarrhea, or heartburn), but hadn't felt enough of a difference in her depression at that level, I had her slowly increase the amount she took until she was up to 3 g a day (1 g with a meal, 3 times a day). She had continual improvement over several weeks, and in two months her depression was gone.

Her sleeping problem disappeared, and as her pains abated, Mary started exercising again. Exercise alone is good for your mood, as well as your physical health, so Mary was getting compound interest on her initial investment. As she felt stronger, impressed by how much better she was feeling, she decided she would give up coffee after all, and felt as good as she could ever remember feeling.

After four months, I told Mary she could try re-introducing foods she had been avoiding into her diet to see what she could tolerate. She did well on a diet more balanced between carbohydrates and protein, as long as she stuck to whole grains and steered clear of refined foods. Even wheat in moderate quantities didn't seem to disagree with her. When she went back to coffee, however, she began to feel depressed again. But as Ida Rolf, the originator of the body mechanics technique known as Rolfing, said to me, you never fall back as far as you were before. Mary caught herself feeling like her old miserable self again and didn't like it, so she tempered the amount of coffee she drank, which enabled her to return to her good mood.

As Mary's mood improved, she decided she wanted to try therapy to work through some of the issues that had been bothering her. She had traveled quite a distance to see me, and so she chose a therapist closer to her home. She reported that she had loved focusing on ways to be her own woman and not live so much in the shadow of her prominent husband. She'd taken a seat on the board of the local animal shelter and started a visiting program at the community hospital, in addition to her work with the PTA, and got a boost from using her talents in new ways. To me, it sounded like she was building up some of her take-charge Warrior traits, a balance that is good for most Stoics.

Mary was pleased with the changes she saw in herself and credited the

Type	General Traits	Beneficial Aspects	Harmful Aspects	Vulnerabilities
Stoics	Dependable	Think of others before	Can't say "no."	Stoics in trouble
	Selfless	themselves.	Bottle up emotions.	tend to get
	Organized	Get stuff done.	Lack self-confidence.	depressed,
	Uncomplaining	Make the world	Don't cry until the	though they
	Considerate	go round.	pain is intense.	generally hide
	Calm	Solder on through	Ignore their own	it well.
	Friendly	hardship.	needs.	
	Even keeled	Have a strong sense	Suppress their anger.	
	Capable	of duty.	Take on too much.	
	Giving	Are good in a crisis.	Feel guilt over	
		Don't place much	whatever they	
		stock in material	don't do.	
		things.	Don't ask for help.	
		Are the salt of the	Avoid conflict at	
		earth.	all costs.	
		Can count Abraham		
		Lincoln as one of		
		their own.		

combination of good nutrition and new behavioral strategies. She felt physically well, and her long-standing depression lifted, and for those reasons she knew she was on the right path. But she said she knew she was really in balance when she discovered she could drink a cup of coffee or two without it bothering her (*and* she didn't feel the need to drink more than that)!

Dietary Guidelines

The easiest way to be the best Stoic you can be is to eat right for your type. To maximize your innate positive tendencies and minimize the potential drawbacks of your type, as a Stoic you should follow a high-protein diet that is relatively high in calories, moderate in fat (with more dairy than meat fat), and low in refined carbohydrates. The more balanced your body is, the less strict you'll need to be with your diet. The supplements described in the next section, along with the mind/body techniques at the end of the chapter, are valuable, but must be built upon a strong foundation of healthful eating.

Essential Foods	Danger Foods
Serotonin-promoting foods such as avocados, walnuts, bananas, pineapple, eggplant, plums, and tomatoes.	Caffeine (though in small amounts and not daily, caffeine is actually positive for most Stoics).

The high-protein, relatively high-calorie diet I recommended to Mary would benefit most Stoics. Reducing refined carbohydrates and cutting out the "whites"—white sugar, white flour, white oils—keep blood sugar and the accompanying mood swings under control, whether or not you have diagnosable hypoglycemia. Of course, the general dietary recommendations covered in Chapter 9 also apply—watch your fat intake, eat organic as much as possible, focus on vegetables, fruits, and whole grains, eat a lot of raw fruits and salad vegetables—and whatever you do, do it in moderation.

You do have to watch the amount of fat in your diet, particularly as you emphasize protein—many meat and dairy sources of protein are also loaded with fat. Besides being a good way to get overweight, overeating of fats contributes to a well-known wide range of serious health problems, from heart disease to diabetes to cancer. There's evidence that fat consumption also contributes to depression. An international study showed that suicide rates are highest in countries where people eat the most fat, particularly from meats. That's particularly remarkable because the researchers showed that suicide rates did not vary according to total calories only, nor with the amount of protein, nor with the level of consumption of alcohol or other stimulants.

The best thing for Stoics (and everyone else) to do right away when they start feeling down is to limit carbohydrates and processed foods in favor of high-quality, low-fat protein and whole, unprocessed, natural foods (either cleaning up their diet for the first time or getting back on the bandwagon if they've fallen off). Strictly avoiding all manufactured foods—refined flour, refined sugar, white (refined) rice—is important because malnutrition

Case in Point

Larry, an executive VP at a large corporation, came to me complaining of chronic depression related to his addiction to coffee and caffeine. He told me he had to have it regularly to feel good. He even used caffeine pills sometimes to get his "hit." Yet when he kept taking it, it eventually made him depressed. Then he'd cut out caffeine and be thrown into complete apathy to the point where he couldn't work. His love/hate relationship with caffeine was a thoroughly entrenched, vicious cycle.

Coffee and tea—caffeine, really—can act as mild antidepressants, and it isn't uncommon to find people self-medicating with them, just as Larry was (and Mary from earlier in the chapter). But as my colleague Serafina Corsello once told me, if you use it and abuse it, you lose it. The body will rebel against excesses of things that, in moderate amounts, you could probably enjoy your whole life without a problem. That's what happened to Larry: He'd become intolerant, and his body reacted to it now as if it were allergic. Anyone who uses caffeine as a drug will probably become intolerant.

I advised Larry to start taking thiamine (vitamin B1), which caffeine depletes. I also recommended a basic panel of general vitamin and mineral supplements, because coffee interferes with digestion and can impair the absorption of nutrients from food. (Stoics with hypoglycemia should note that coffee interferes with the digestion of protein in particular.)

But my most emphatic advice to Larry was to strike a truce with coffee, drinking it in moderation and using the minimum he needed. Sure enough, through trial and error, he discovered that if he kept it to one or two cups of coffee a day, he felt good. When it dragged to three or four cups, he cut it out entirely until he could go back to just one or two cups. With a well-nourished body, that's all he needed to maintain both his good spirits and top performance on the job.

from poor eating habits is most likely the biochemical trigger of your depression. All these refined foods are guaranteed to malnourish you if you use them steadily in your diet. Refined sugar is especially bad because its concentrated energy isn't balanced by necessary nutrients—they've been stripped away in the refining process. That sends your blood sugar on a roller-coaster ride, which will eventually wear out your pancreas and cause dramatic mood swings in the meantime.

Coffee and tea (caffeine) can act as mild antidepressants, though caffeine is a bit of a hot potato. In moderation (and not on a regular basis), some Stoics can use caffeine for an occasional boost without any negative effects. Even better is a cup of warm milk, or a small serving of turkey, which contains tryptophan. A dish of whole wheat pasta can have a similar effect, increasing the amount of tryptophan reaching the brain. Your body converts tryptophan, a natural sedative and sleeping aid, into serotonin. Other foods that boost serotonin include avocados, walnuts, bananas, tomatoes, eggplant, plums, and pineapple.

The Stoic Diet

The Stoic diet is not about counting calories (though with exercise, you will also maintain a healthy weight and general good health on this diet). It is more like the FDA Food Pyramid (which has its flaws) in focusing on the number of servings of different kinds of foods that Stoics should build into their daily diets. The Stoic diet should consist of:

- 5–7 small meals a day
- 2–3 servings dairy protein
- 1–2 servings meat protein
- 5–8 servings vegetables
- 2–3 servings fruit
- 4–5 servings whole grains
- 2 servings legumes
- 1 serving nuts and seeds (optional)

FOOD	BEST CHOICES	GOOD CHOICES	AVOID
Dairy Protein (2–3 servings)	raw milk cottage cheese yogurt cheddar cheese	pasteurized milk	homogenized milk in clear plastic containers canned, powdered milk
Meat Protein (1–2 servings)	sardines chicken (enriched with DHA) eggs (enriched with DHA) salmon turkey herring halibut	poultry red meat eggs (not enriched with DHA) fish caviar pork tuna	canned, processed, and frozen meats with preservatives
Vegetables (5–8 servings)	avocados eggplant tomatoes seaweed (hijiki, nori, and kombu) peas alfalfa sprouts broccoli cabbage carrots potatoes spinach asparagus lettuce onions cauliflower	Brussels sprouts collards kale mustard greens parsley peppers mushrooms iceberg lettuce	canned and frozen vegetables, especially with EDTA, preservatives, or additives
Fruit (2–3 servings)	bananas pineapple plums lemons cantaloupe oranges	apricots berries melons cherries limes guava grapefruit kiwi mangoes papaya strawberries	canned fruit, especially in rich sugar syrups

FOOD	BEST CHOICES	GOOD CHOICES	AVOID
Whole Grains (4–5 servings)	whole-grain bread whole-grain cereal brown rice shredded wheat cereal whole wheat oatmeal		white bread white rice white flour
Legumes (2 servings)	tofu black beans pinto beans garbanzo beans (chickpeas) lentils navy beans lima beans soybeans	canned beans frozen beans	canned and frozen beans with added sugar, EDTA, hydrogenated oil, or preservatives
Nuts and Seeds (1 serving, optional)	peanuts almonds sunflower seeds walnuts Brazil nuts	pistachios cashews pumpkin seeds (and other squash seeds) pecans sesame seeds	unsalted raw nuts
Sweeteners	maple syrup	honey	white sugar
Beverages	milk green tea (decaffeinated) ginseng tea tomato juice		caffeinated drinks (including coffee, tea, sodas, and diet sodas)
Condiments and Seasonings	brewer's yeast lecithin		yeast

The previous table points out the best specific food choices for Stoics, as well as some foods that should be avoided. Foods not mentioned are basically neutral and you can eat them freely, as long as you have already included plenty of the "best" and "good" choices in your diet.

Blood Chemistry Markers: Neurotransmitters

The Stoic in trouble typically has low serotonin, high blood cortisol, high histamines, low zinc and magnesium, and high copper levels. Testing for these substances can help confirm a diagnosis and point to the best treatments. Discuss them with your doctor. (For details about these tests, see "The Workup" on page 124, in Chapter 4: The Guardian.)

SEROTONIN

Low serotonin in the brain is well established as a sign of depression and is widely accepted by neuropsychiatric scientists. Serotonin in the blood correlates well with brain serotonin levels, so we can test for blood levels of this neurotransmitter. The most popular prescription antidepressants (Prozac, Paxil, and Zoloft) work by keeping serotonin levels up. (These SSRIs, or selective serotonin reuptake inhibitors, work by preventing the absorption and breakdown of serotonin, leaving it available for the body to use.) There's a wide range of "normal" levels for serotonin, so you obviously can't consider the results in a vacuum. But serotonin correlates very nicely with mood: When serotonin increases, mood improves, and when serotonin decreases, depression closes in. Your readings will vary according to your mood at the time, even if you are in good balance. If you suspect that you are a Stoic in trouble, your doctor will probably want to test your serotonin level to confirm a biochemical source for your depression and to evaluate the extent of the imbalance.

HISTAMINE

The test for histamine levels is harder to come by. A few research scientists have accepted high histamines as a marker for depression, but few clinicians

Normal Levels for Brain Chemistry Markers	
Serotonin	55–260 ng/ml (nanograms per milliliter)
Histamine	9–141 ng/ml
Cortisol	levels vary during the day: 8–26 mg/100 ml in the morning; 2–18 mg/100 ml in the afternoon; < 6 mg/100 ml at midnight.
Zinc	60–130 mcg/dl
Copper	65–155 mcg/dl (micrograms per deciliter) (normal range varies from lab to lab)
Magnesium	1.7–2.5 mg/dl

focus on it. Serotonin has stolen histamine's thunder, taking over as the current "it" neurotransmitter. And, in a sad illustration of how unscientific medical reasoning can be, checking histamine has slipped even further under the radar recently in part because the major proponent of its clinical use died. Over the years, it's gotten harder and harder to get an accurate test from the commercial labs.

It is often worth the effort to get histamine tested through a specialized lab, however, as there is a simple and specific treatment for a high-histamine depression. Calcium and the amino acid d-1-methionine, at 500 mg each, twice a day, can lower histamine levels and reverse depression. One good option is to do a histamine test only if a serotonin test does not provide useful results. Different labs use different units to measure histamine levels, but all of them send back test results with the range considered normal and information on whether your result falls above or below that range.

Because serotonin and histamine both might not be off in any given case of depression, checking both can be helpful, especially in more complicated cases. Even without the help of a lab, there are a few clues our bodies give us regarding serotonin and histamine levels. In depression resulting from high histamine levels, people are generally very sober, sad, gray, and obviously depressed. (*Low* histamines cause different sorts of mental disturbances all together, including, potentially, mania and even hallucinations.) A depressed person with high histamine levels will *appear* depressed. This is not the "smiling depression" that so many Stoics in trouble fall victim to. High histamine levels have even been associated with suicide risk.

CORTISOL

The adrenal hormone cortisol is another marker used by researchers, and can be tested commercially. Studies have shown that cortisol levels are twice as high in severely depressed people than in non-depressed people—and that the cortisol returns to a normal level after treatment and recovery. In fact, lowering cortisol levels is one indicator that treatment is working. One study showed nearly half of patients hospitalized for depression had extremely elevated cortisol levels, compared to just 6 percent of other hospitalized patients. I do want to note, however, that in some cases of depression, cortisol may be *low*. That would result in a more chronic though probably less severe depression, associated with a worn-out or burned-out feeling, fatigue, and hopelessness.

Cortisol indicates a general stress reaction. Any kind of stress will raise it, so it doesn't indicate depression specifically, the way serotonin does. So you might have a cortisol reading that is way up there because you are depressed, or because of an overwhelming life problem. It might be up because you are scheduled to have surgery, or because you just started a new job with many more responsibilities, or any of the other myriad reasons you might be experiencing high levels of stress.

It's the stress you want to get rid of, not the cortisol per se. The cortisol is there for a reason. In fact, during the Cuban Missile Crisis, President Kennedy received injections of adrenocorticotropic hormone (ACTH) to raise his cortisol to help him cope with the extreme stress he was experiencing. Addison's disease, which he suffered from, is a deficiency in the body of the production of cortisol. Your body can't continuously produce large amounts of cortisol without wearing out the system, however, so you do want to manage your stress as much as possible.

I personally don't order this test regularly as a diagnostic tool, since the results are informative but not particularly useful. But I'm mentioning it here because you may be able to get your cortisol levels tested—and because high cortisol *is* strongly linked to depression. In fact, severe mental states, including clinical depression, result in the highest cortisol levels known to exist—higher even than if you had a tumor in the adrenal gland (where cortisol is produced). I look at it as further proof of just how inseparable "mind" and "body" are, and how *all* medicine must be "mind/body" medicine to be fully effective.

MAGNESIUM

Magnesium is important in many chemical functions in the body, especially in relation to the nervous system. Studies show that depressed people have low magnesium levels—lower than "normal," and lower than in non-depressed people. One international study showed higher rates of depression and suicide in certain counties where magnesium is generally deficient in the local diet. A shortage of magnesium can also cause insomnia, which can contribute to or worsen depression.

Low magnesium can cause depression, and depression can lower magnesium levels, but either way, supplementing should help reverse the depression. (Even if you don't use a supplement, when depression lifts, magnesium levels rise.)

COPPER

Copper deficiency is associated with lethargic depression—mineral deficiencies in general cause people to look really passive and malnourished. But much more common is depression connected to *high* levels of copper, and that kind of depression usually involves a "racing mind" and severe agitation. Copper is a brain stimulant, and high copper is basically too much of a good thing, in the same way caffeine can be. You feel terrible, over-excited, and burnt out.

One way to see the toxic effects of excess copper is to look at what happens to people with Wilson's disease, a genetic enzymatic malfunction that causes the body to absorb too much copper. The eventual cause of death in Wilson's disease is liver failure, but before that point, the extremely high copper levels cause mental illness and even psychosis. Here, though, we're talking about much less severe poisonings—just imbalances, really, which manifest as overexcitement, insomnia, or depression.

ZINC

Low zinc produces the same kind of effect as high copper, since zinc is a sedative that must be in balance with copper for stable mental health. Because it is so important that the ratio between the two is balanced, low zinc can make even a normal copper level act like a toxic high copper.

Stress raises copper and lowers zinc, creating or exacerbating an imbalance between the two, which is one way stress contributes to depression. If your copper level is high, try to lower the amount in your diet (avoid mushrooms, shellfish, coffee, and chocolate) and the amount you get from environmental exposure (see "The Great Water Cop(per) Out" below), and take zinc to rebalance the proportions.

We need trace amounts of copper to be healthy, but we get a lot of copper from our environment and get overloaded without realizing it. Copper is used in fungicides and insecticides, which is just one of the reasons the

---

The Great Water Cop(per) Out

If you live in a newly built home or have recently replaced pipes, don't drink the first water out of your pipes in the morning. Run the water for a few minutes to flush out the water that's been sitting there overnight (with plenty of time to soak up copper from your pipes) before you ingest any. As long as you get those slight green stains around your drains (if you have white sinks and tubs) or as long as your water has the telltale bitter taste of copper, you're getting too much of it in your water. After a few years, depending on how hard or soft your water is, the pipes get coated with calcium, which stops the copper from leaching into the water, and it is fine to drink even the first water of the day. Before then, distilling water will take out the copper.

Heavy Metal Poisoning

One of the first signs of heavy metal poisoning is depression, so a Stoic in trouble—or anyone who is depressed—should wonder if they are being poisoned by something in their environment. The brain is the organ most sensitive to chemicals, and mental symptoms are often the first sign of physical illness.

Lead poisoning is no doubt to blame for many cases of depression and for severity of symptoms. Depression sets in before the most drastic neurological and psychiatric effects, such as retardation and lowered IQ appear. The brain has only a few ways of letting us know it is not working properly, and depression is one of the first flares sent up. Though lead levels in gas and paint are now famously regulated, other sources, like jet fuel, still pour lead into our world.

Hair analysis is a good way to screen for heavy metal exposure, despite its flaws in other areas. This test is affordable and non-invasive. Blood or urine tests would be appropriate to follow up on any results showing high levels of lead. Short of that, you can make some educated guesses about your risk. People living in urban environments, for example, are exposed to more lead than those living in rural areas. The more time you spend around cars and industry, the more lead your body absorbs.

In an ideal world, we'd have zero tolerance for lead in the human body. Officially, there is no level that is "good." Practically speaking, however, noticeable problems don't show up until blood lead is more than 80 mcg/100 ml. Officially, 100 mcg/100 ml means lead poisoning.

The connection between mercury and mental illness has been known for a long time. The Mad Hatter in *Alice in Wonderland* was instantly recognizable to original readers, because hatters, who

(continued)

Heavy Metal Poisoning *(continued)*

handled mercury freely in making felt hats, absorbed considerable amounts of mercury through their skin that they really were "mad"—thus the phrase "mad as a hatter," and Lewis Carroll's play on it.

I've heard enough about the dangers of mercury to make me concerned about the stuff in my teeth: "Silver" fillings are almost 50 percent mercury. You have to wonder: Why put a poison in your mouth? I've treated chronic depression sufferers who claimed that they felt better after they had their silver-mercury amalgam fillings removed and replaced with gold or ceramic. I learned a less drastic technique in Germany: Swishing olive oil around your mouth in the morning grabs up the mercury coming out of fillings (studies show most comes out early in the day). The best alternative is to take the best care of your teeth you can, and choose ceramic or gold fillings when you do have to deal with a cavity.

The better nourished you are, the less likely your body is to absorb toxins like lead and mercury. But if you are deficient in the metals normally found in the body—like calcium, magnesium, copper, zinc, manganese, chromium, and selenium—your body will try to use heavy metals in their place. That's one more reason to follow the healthy eating principles presented in Chapter 9.

pesticides you get with any non-organic produce are bad for you (and why you must thoroughly scrub and peel your fruits and vegetables unless they are organic). Mostly our bodies are copper toxic thanks to the traces our water absorbs from our plumbing. Pipes are copper now, which is an improvement over lead, but we're still getting too much of a heavy metal in our water. High intelligence is associated with high copper levels (and high zinc—a balance), and kids with high copper levels do better in school. But the amount of copper many people absorb is too much of a good thing.

There's enough strong evidence about the link between the minerals zinc, copper, and magnesium and depression that all psychiatrists should be testing for them. But they aren't. Testing for these minerals can give you important insight into your condition and can point the way toward possible treatments. If your doctor doesn't suggest the test, you should.

Natural Medicine Solutions

To support the proper diet—and provide backup to an imperfect diet—each type should take certain daily supplements. Beyond that, I'll cover interventions for Stoics-in-trouble—still natural approaches, but bigger guns (or, in some cases, bigger doses of daily supplements).

Malnutrition—poor eating habits, no matter what the reason or other effects on the body—can cause depression. Specific deficiencies in several vitamins have been associated with depression, including vitamin C, and the B vitamins folic acid, thiamine (B1), cobalamin (B12), pyridoxine (B6), pantothenic acid (B5) and riboflavin (B2). We'll look first at the effects of these deficiencies, and then at correcting the imbalance with supplements. Finally, we'll continue with additional supplements.

Because the range of normal is so wide for these vitamins, and because individuals vary so much in their needs for them—depending on their general physiology and on how much stress they are under at any given time—it isn't practical to test for them as an indicator of depression. If you are depressed, it's good to assume that you are not getting what you need in the way of vitamin C and the B vitamins. Even if you are in the "normal" range for those vitamins, that level may not be enough for you. I've said it before, and I'll say it again: Normal does not mean optimal.

DAILY SUPPLEMENTS

Used daily, these vitamins and minerals are meant to correct deficiencies. However, I use them at higher doses to make use of the full range of their benefits. They are not magic pills! They are meant to be used in conjunction with a diet well balanced for your particular type, which will support and

Daily Supplements

(Start with lower doses and increase as necessary for desired effect.)

Riboflavin (vitamin B2): 100 mg

Niacin (vitamin B3): 100–3000 mg

Pantothenic acid (vitamin B5): 500 mg

Pyridoxine (vitamin B6): 100 mg

Folic acid: 1 mg

Cobalamin (vitamin B12): 100 mg

Thiamine (vitamin B1): 50–100 mg

Vitamin C: 500–3000 mg

Zinc: 0–30 mg

Magnesium: 0–500 mg

DHA: up to 1250 mg

boost the effects. Where there is a range of doses, use the lower levels for prevention, or maintenance, and higher levels when you need a therapeutic effect (when you are out of balance or in trouble). As always, take only what you need.

B Vitamins

Deficiencies in several other B vitamins, including pyridoxine (B6), riboflavin (B2), thiamine (B1), and cobalamin (B12), are also associated with depression, though the studies are not as numerous as the ones investigating folic acid. Considering that all the B vitamins are essential for optimal brain function, there's more than enough evidence to convince me that a B-complex supplement is necessary for my Stoic patients, both in balance and in trouble.

Folic Acid A deficiency in folic acid, a B vitamin sometimes called folate, lowers serotonin levels and decreases SAMe (a substance that raises serotonin, as we'll discuss in a later section of this chapter). As a result, there's been a lot of research examining its role in depression. We know that de-

What's in a B complex?

Thiamine (vitamin B1)

Riboflavin (vitamin B2)

Niacin (niacinamide) (vitamin B3)

Calcium pantothenate (pantothenic acid) (vitamin B5)

Pyridoxine (vitamin B6)

Cobalamin (vitamin B12)

Folic acid (folacin, folate)

Choline

Inositol

Biotin

PABA (para aminobenzoic acid)

pression is a common symptom of folic acid deficiency and that people with major depression have lower folic acid levels than those who are not depressed. Additionally, the lower your folate level is, the deeper your depression is likely to be, the less likely you are to be successful with treatment, and the longer you're likely to stay depressed.

People with a folic acid deficiency being treated for depression with pharmaceuticals responded better to the drugs when they were also given folic acid supplements, compared to those who used only the drugs. Patients given supplements got better quicker and were more likely to make a full recovery. The association between folic acid deficiency and depression strengthens with age, so the older you are, the more important this link should be to you. Folic acid deficiency may also cause fatigue, so if you experience fatigue along with depression, you may find supplements to be particularly beneficial.

Folic acid deficiency interferes with the synthesis of serotonin, causing serotonin levels in the brain to fall, leading to, or worsening, depression. Along with pyridoxine (vitamin B6) and cobalamin (vitamin B12), folic acid is one of the most common deficiencies in depressed people. Supplements of this B vitamin are helpful to some Stoics in trouble, particularly those who also have insomnia, or are forgetful, irritable, or apathetic.

Good brain function requires sufficient folic acid. Folic acid helps prevent and reverse hypoglycemia. It works with vitamin B12 in the neurological system.

Although 200–500 mcg a day (which you can get from food) is enough to make a difference, studies using high doses available only by prescription (15–50 mg) have shown folic acid to perform as well as drugs. However, large doses require close medical supervision, since high levels are potentially toxic, and because of the complicated relationship between folic acid and cobalamin (vitamin B12). Large amounts of folic acid can mask a deficiency in B12, until irreversible nerve and brain damage may occur. If you do take folic acid supplements, you should always take B12 as well for that reason. I usually recommend that the B12 be given by injection for better absorption.

Early on in my practice, folic acid was widely available in 10-mg tablets, and I frequently used orthomolecular doses of 1–2 tablets (and sometimes

---

Folic Acid

RDA: 200 mcg (However, even conservative mainstream recommendations now call for at least 400 mcg a day, particularly for women of childbearing age, as sufficient folic acid is necessary for the prevention of neural tube birth defects.)

Recommended dose (in balance): 800 mcg–2 mg daily

Recommended dose (in trouble): 1–40 mg daily with cobalamin (B12) and zinc

Maximum safe level: Unknown. Levels of 40–60 mg a day have been used without toxicity.

Contraindications: If you are taking epileptic medications, consult your doctor before taking folic acid.

up to 4) a day to good effect in many stubborn cases of depression. (Folic acid in these larger doses also is often a memory enhancer, and theoretically many be good for Alzheimer's disease and other neurodegenerative diseases.) Folic acid is now restricted, available only in 20-mg tablets by prescription or up to 400 mcg (a microgram is just 1/1000 of a milligram) over the counter, even though it has in recent years become more widely known as crucial for preventing neural tube birth defects.

Folic acid was never a first-line treatment, but a significant number of people respond to it when nothing else works. With your doctor's prescription, you can obtain higher dose (20 mg) folic acid tablets from special compounding pharmacies. The studies showing the usefulness of larger doses corroborate my clinical experience, but I haven't been able to use the orthomolecular doses much since the restrictions were put in place in the early 1980s. Some people benefit from just the 1-mg dose, so it may be worth trying if your other options don't do the trick.

Niacin (Vitamin B3) Niacin is a necessary cog in the serotonin-producing machinery, and it is often effective in depression when taken with a high-protein diet. If I had to choose only one vitamin for my repertoire for improving mood or guarding against the blues, this is the one I'd probably pick. Niacin, sometimes known as nicotinic acid or niacinamide, and occasionally as vitamin B3, raises serotonin levels no matter what's causing them to drop—impending divorce or chronic malnutrition. Taking niacin, an all-important coenzyme, allows the body to use all its tryptophan to boost serotonin rather than divert some of it to make niacin. Together with all the B vitamins, niacin also improves cerebral circulation. Insufficient niacin can cause depression.

Niacin is one of the least expensive vitamins. Therapeutic doses cost only pennies a day. It is without side effects when used correctly, and treats the cause of the problem, not just the symptoms. All at about one-fiftieth of the price of drugs like Prozac. As a kind of bonus, niacin also lowers cholesterol, helping prevent heart disease.

Taking niacin in orthomolecular doses will help lift your depression, even if your levels are normal to begin with. Of course, those who need it most urgently are those who have an actual deficiency. In my experience, for people with depression and niacin deficiency, life seems terrible, and they often express their distress in a "tearful depression" (somewhat less common in Stoics than "smiling depression"). They experience everything as if through a veil of tears. I've seen many weepy patients like that who start taking niacin, usually in combination with a B-complex supplement, and a couple of weeks later come in pulled together. They are frequently relieved to find their problems to be a reflection of a faulty outlook from faulty chemistry rather than from a fixed condition or personality defect.

In most people, insufficient niacin causes depression or inability to concentrate. Even mild cases can cause apathy, mental fatigue, gloominess, foggy thinking, anger, irritability, weakness, and sleepiness. Niacin deficiency can also make you feel fearful, apprehensive, suspicious, alienated,

---

Niacin

RDA (men): 18 mg
   (women): 13 mg

Recommended dose (in balance): for men: 100 mg daily
                             for women: 60 mg daily

Recommended dose (in trouble): 500–3,000 mg daily

Maximum safe level: Any dose that does not cause diarrhea, vomiting, or bowel upset is safe. If you take more than 3,000 mg (3 g), you must have a physician monitoring you.

Contraindications: Do not take niacin if you are taking high blood pressure medication, as it could make your pressure drop too low. Don't take it if you have ulcers, gout, active liver disease, or a liver disorder. Since niacin raises blood sugar, people with diabetes should consult their doctors about managing their insulin dose before taking niacin. Niacinamide can cause dark spots on the skin.

reclusive, and excessively worried. It may give you insomnia. In some cases, it can even interfere with moral sensibilities, leading to behaviors like thoughtless promiscuity, pathological lying, or petty thievery.

Niacin helps the thought processes remain realistic and less influenced by the primitive emotional brain. Feeling worried or sad is not a problem if there is an actual cause for it. We need those emotions to survive and to be fully human. But when the primitive brain hijacks too much control because of poor neurotransmitter communication, you can get those feelings and all those listed above *without* any reality-based cause. *That's* a problem.

Because we rely so heavily on highly refined high-carbohydrate food, niacin deficiency is widespread in America. Like most B vitamins, niacin is required for carbohydrate metabolism, so the large amounts of sugars and starches in many processed foods divert niacin needed for other functions. Furthermore, even in some foods rich in niacin, like corn, it occurs in a form that sometimes the human body can't make use of. So even when we eat niacin-rich foods, we may not always get enough of it.

Niacin raises blood sugar, so it is helpful in hypoglycemia. And it is crucial in making neurotransmitters involved in moods.

To raise serotonin and treat depression, I prescribe 500–3,000 mg of niacin a day, starting with lower doses and gradually increasing. Niacin works best with a high-protein diet (like the one recommended for all Stoics) and should be taken with meals. Like all vitamins, it works in conjunction with many other nutrients in foods. Also, since it is a weak acid, taking it with food lessens the possibility of it upsetting your stomach.

Some people experience an unpleasant "niacin flush" (like a hot flash, the body feels hot, and sweats, and the face reddens) at higher doses, because niacin releases histamine, which causes a powerful dilation of the surface blood vessels. But that shouldn't bother most people. Many people just seem not to be prone to it, and some people actually rather enjoy the sensation, or at least don't mind it at all. Try beginning with just 100 mg three times a day, and building up from there to find the point where you see benefits but don't trigger that annoying side effect. If you get a flush that does bother you, stopping niacin will make it go away. Lowering the dose might also work. More expensive buffered niacin is sold as "flushless" because attaching it to another B vitamin prevents that effect. Those options provide the same mood benefits, though they do not lower blood cholesterol the way niacin does. You could also try taking niacin with a cold drink to suppress the flush. (*Don't* take it with a hot drink—or just before a hot

Case in Point

Susanna seemed to have everything to live for. She was a young college student, friendly, and attractive. If it weren't for the fact that she told me she was sometimes suicidal, I would have had a hard time believing she was depressed when we first met because of the peppy way she presented herself. If I had harbored any doubts, her lab tests would have put them to rest: She had a very low blood serotonin level.

Susanna thought she had a pretty good diet, but when I pressed her for details, it became clear that she was eating a lot of sugar and some junk food, and she wasn't getting much protein. I encouraged her to add more cheese, beans, meat, and fish to her regular diet, along with plenty of vegetables, fruits, and whole grains. I also advised her to cut out white sugar and white flour.

At the same time, I started her on 3 g of niacin a day, along with a multivitamin and -mineral supplement to make sure she would get at least the minimum levels of what her body needed. The niacin was key because it is an important precursor to tryptophan, which in turn is converted into serotonin in the body. The other supplements were aimed at making sure the niacin would have what it needed to work efficiently. (Incidentally, Susanna was not taking any prescription antidepressants.)

Within six weeks, Susanna was no longer depressed. I repeated the serotonin measurement and found quite normal levels.

shower!) Some people use an antihistamine to block the flush reaction if the dose they need to alleviate depression also triggers the flush.

Niacinamide, a metabolite of niacin, can cause liver damage in high concentrations. So if you take this form, do not use more than 1500 mg (1.5 g) a day. For the same reason, you need to be monitored if you take niacin along with any statin drug.

Pyridoxine (Vitamin B6) The body uses pyridoxine (vitamin B6) in the production of several neurotransmitters, including noradrenaline, dopamine, and serotonin. Deficiencies in any of those neurotransmitters can cause mood problems. To take just one example, insufficient amounts of B6 may mean insufficient serotonin, and as we've already discussed, low serotonin leads to depression. Vitamin B6 is also a crucial coenzyme for marking monoamine (MAO) neurotransmitters, which are, in turn, important in maintaining a mellow mood. (MAO inhibitors, which are used to treat depression, may cause a deficiency in vitamin B6.) Vitamin B6 levels are, in fact, low in most depressed people.

B6 levels are also low in women taking The Pill or HRT, perhaps accounting for the mood problems sometimes associated with those drugs. But taking B6 supplements to correct the deficiency can get rid of all those symptoms. Anyone with a deficiency should benefit from supplements, but

---

Pyridoxine (Vitamin B6)

RDA (men): 2 mg daily
    (women): 1–6 mg daily

Recommended dose (in balance): 10–50 mg daily

Recommended dose (in trouble): 100–1,000 mg daily

Contraindications: If you're taking L-dopa (as for Parkinson's disease), check with a doctor before using vitamin B6 supplements.

studies show that women on The Pill who are also low in B6 received the greatest and most rapid results.

Vitamin B6 is required to make tryptophan into serotonin. MAO inhibitor drugs can cause a B6 deficiency, so taking a supplement is advisable if you use them. Take doses above 1,000 mg only with magnesium.

Cobalamin (Vitamin B12) Lack of cobalamin (vitamin B12) can cause depression even three to five years before it is severe enough to cause anemia. B12 levels are lower in depressed people than non-depressed people, on average, and deficiency is thirty times more common in patients hospitalized for depression than in the general population, according to one study. Even if your B12 level isn't low enough to qualify technically as a deficiency, it can still cause problems: In one study, the lower the level of B12, the poorer the score on various tests of mental health—although every patient fell within "normal" levels.

Vitamin B12 is crucial for growth and maintenance of nerve cells—including the brain. It is good for fighting stress, fatigue, and insomnia, all of which often occur in conjunction with depression. A balance of B12 and folic acid may work most efficiently to relieve depression (another reason for taking a B-complex vitamin rather than a supplement of a single B vitamin).

Cobalamin (Vitamin B12)

RDA: 6 mcg daily (taken orally)

Recommended Dose (in balance): 1000 mcg daily (taken orally or sublingually)

Recommended Dose (in trouble): 1000 mcg by injection every 2–3 days for 2–3 months

Maximum safe level: Unknown

Contraindications: None

In another study, the percentage of hospitalized mental patients with low B12 levels was thirty times higher than in the general population, which underlines the importance of B12 to good brain function. Without enough of it, you may experience confusion, memory loss—even hallucinations, delusions, and paranoia, in the most extreme cases.

Thiamine (Vitamin B1)   Thiamine (vitamin B1), an antioxidant, is also often low in cases of depression. Depression is a common symptom of thiamine deficiency—and so is irritability. Those two are a very popular combination in the patients I see, and I always recommend a B-complex supplement and sometimes an additional dose of thiamine. If depression comes with a component of apathy or anxiety, I again think thiamine. Thiamine is intimately involved with carbohydrate metabolism, and carbohydrate metabolism is what provides the fuel for our bodies, so fatigue is another hallmark of thiamine deficiency–related depression. If you find you are exhausted after jogging just a block or two, for example, make sure you are getting sufficient thiamine.

Thiamine is used in energy metabolism, in the workings of the nervous system, and in repairing cells. Research shows that thiamine improves brain functioning even in a normal brain, and those whose brain chemistry is out of balance definitely benefit. In one study, people reported being more clearheaded, composed, and energetic after taking thiamine supplements for two months—and their original thiamine levels were considered adequate by conventional standards.

Many of the substances that depressed people sometimes self-medicate with—alcohol, caffeine, and junk food prime among them—create thiamine deficiency, leading to a downward spiral. Prolonged heavy alcohol use destroys the stomach's ability to absorb thiamine and other nutrients. Caffeine also interferes with thiamine and protein absorption (but to a lesser extent than alcohol). Metabolizing refined flour and sugar requires thiamine. But thiamine is one of the important nutrients largely lost in the refining process, so eating refined (incomplete) foods creates a deficit in your body. The steady American diet of refined foods provides the calories

> ## Thiamine (Vitamin B1)
>
> **RDA:** 1.5 mg
>
> **Recommended dose (in balance):** 0–100 mg daily
>
> **Recommended dose (in trouble):** 100–500 mg twice daily, up to 500–1,000 mg twice daily orally, but only under the guidance of a health care professional.
>
> **Maximum safe level:** It is not necessary to take more than 1–2 grams a day, which is known to be safe.
>
> **Contraindications:** None.

our bodies demand but without the thiamine it needs to convert those calories into energy, because processing destroys thiamine. Tobacco, alcohol, and caffeine also burn thiamine we can't afford to lose. Raw fish, clams, and oysters also contain an enzyme that destroys thiamine, so you should eat them in moderation or increase your intake of thiamine.

Thiamine supplements can be helpful for depression. When you take it orally, only about one percent of it is absorbed, so relatively large doses are required to do the trick. Stress—including the stress of exercise—increases the need for thiamine. If exercise exhausts rather than energizes you, you may need more of this vitamin.

Thiamine deficiency can cause depression, along with irritability, apathy, emotional instability, confusion, fatigue, insomnia, headaches, indigestion, occasional diarrhea (but more commonly constipation), poor appetite, weight loss, and feelings of numbness or burning in hands and feet.

Riboflavin (Vitamin B2) Riboflavin (vitamin B2) is also often low in cases of depression. Riboflavin deficiency often goes hand in hand with vitamin B6 deficiency. The greater the deprivation of this nutrient, the deeper the depression. Studies show that people taking antidepressant prescriptions

> ## Riboflavin (Vitamin B2)
>
> RDA: 1.3 mg
>
> Recommended dose (in balance): 10 mg daily
>
> Recommended dose (in trouble): 10–400 mg daily, with balancing B-complex vitamin.
>
> Maximum safe level: Unknown. We only absorb 20 mg at a time, and the rest is excreted.
>
> Contraindications: None.

see more improvement when they take supplements of riboflavin and thiamine (and B6) than do those on antidepressants alone.

Lack of riboflavin can cause depression, since it is a crucial ingredient in converting amino acids into neurotransmitters.

Pantothenic Acid (Vitamin B5) I call vitamin B5 the "antistress vitamin" because it helps strengthen the adrenal glands, which produce the antistress hormone cortisol and the mineral corticoids, which keep up our mineral balance. Deficiency in B5 causes fatigue, insomnia, restlessness, irritability, and depression. It is especially helpful for the combination of fatigue and depression that characterizes low adrenal function in the face of overwhelming stressors like chronic allergies—or just the stress of daily life. If you feel "burnt out," stamina-boosting B5 will be a good choice for you.

B5 works together with the essential fatty acids in eggs or lecithin, vitamin C, sodium, and potassium in supporting the adrenals. Taking supplements of these is required for the best result. (To get the particular essential fatty acids you need to make B5 most effective, eat two eggs or take one tablespoon of lecithin a day.)

If your burnout is due to adrenal exhaustion, you may experience aching in the small of your lower back where your adrenals are located. In bad

> ## Pantothenic Acid (Vitamin B5); Calcium Pantothenate
>
> **RDA:** 10 mg
>
> **Recommended dose (in balance):** 250 mg daily
>
> **Recommended dose (in trouble):** 500 mg–1 g twice daily
>
> **Maximum safe level:** Unknown. It is not necessary to take more than 2 g a day, which is known to be safe.
>
> **Contraindications:** None.

cases, if you press there, it will feel sore. Getting more B5 from your diet or supplements can ease the pain.

Vitamin C

Insufficient vitamin C can also contribute to depression. Vitamin C levels are often lower in depressed people than in their non-depressed peers. In one study, about a third of patients hospitalized for depression had levels below where we know the immune system starts to weaken. Depression is one of the first symptoms of scurvy—the disease resulting from dire lack of vitamin C. Tiredness, irritability, and a general, non-specific feeling of poor health also herald scurvy—or just a lack of vitamin C.

Clinical trials have shown that supplements of vitamin C help lessen depression. Taking vitamin C in the ascorbic acid form can improve the results of lithium therapy by acidifying the body so the drug can provide the same benefit at a lower dose. (Though the studies in this regard tend to use intravenous vitamins, as long as you're getting and absorbing what you need, it shouldn't matter how you receive it.) Vitamin C can also reduce negative side effects of these drugs.

Stress (or depression or emotional distress) burns vitamin C at a rapid rate, causing a dramatic drop in the body's vitamin C level. Since vitamin C lowers excessive adrenaline levels, and adrenaline rises with agitation and anxiety, it is especially important to get enough vitamin C when you are stressed or depressed.

Vitamin C

RDA: 45 mg

Recommended dose (general): 1000–3000 mg

Recommended dose (in trouble): 1000–30,000 mg; use mineral ascorbate to avoid distention.

Maximum safe level: Unknown.

Vitamin C is a painkiller, general antitoxin, and immune-system supporter, as well as an antidepressant. Sufficient levels help prevent depression, and large doses can help eliminate it. Vitamin C crosses the blood/brain barrier only to a limited extent, making large doses necessary to effect even the slighter increases in brain vitamin C we're after. When it does reach the brain in sufficient quantity, it promotes a feeling of well-being. The human body does not make vitamin C—we're almost the only animal that doesn't make our own, with the exception of one type of fruit-eating bat—yet we must have it for good health. A well-rounded diet goes a long way toward that end, but the benefits of large doses require supplements.

Linus Pauling estimated that our ancestors got about 10 g of vitamin C a day in their diet, but we now average about 500 mg a day. I recommend a minimum of 3 g a day for depression, working up from there if necessary. There is no established level of toxicity, so there's no notable risk in taking megadoses. You can get diarrhea by taking too much vitamin C, but this side effect can be eliminated by lowering the dose. Taking vitamin C with food will minimize any potential intestinal discomfort by buffering its acidity (vitamin C is also known as ascorbic acid).

I prescribe niacin and vitamin C in equal measure for most mental conditions, since niacin is a methyl acceptor, soaking up toxic methyl chemicals produced by the adrenal stress reaction. I also recommend mixing powdered vitamin C with citrus juice—which is my own habit—to get the benefit of the bioflavonoids that always accompany vitamin C in nature. You can also take bioflavonoids in tablet form, either separately or in combination with vitamin C. Taking the nutrients as a duo maximizes the effectiveness and efficiency of vitamin C. Bioflavonoids, occasionally referred to as "vitamin P," are most commonly used as a separate supplement to treat easy bruising. In fact, taking large doses of vitamin C over a long period of time without bioflavonoids can *cause* easy bruising. These days, many vitamin C tablets are fortified with bioflavonoids.

Magnesium

Magnesium is a well-known sedative and also has an antidepressant effect no matter what your current levels. A deficiency, however, can show up as irritability and depression. Magnesium can also help you sleep better. I recommend chelated magnesium, because the body absorbs it better, at 400 mg a day. In some people, magnesium has a laxative effect, but the chelated form makes that less likely. (Lowering your dose should eliminate that if it is a problem.)

Magnesium

RDA: 6 mg daily

Recommended dose (general): 400 mg daily (chelated form)

Recommended dose (in trouble): 600 mg daily

Maximum safe level: Unknown; don't take more than 600 mg daily

Contraindications: Low blood pressure

Zinc

To keep copper in balance, and for a whole host of reasons, zinc is important for Stoics. Liquid zinc is the form best absorbed by the body, but it can be difficult to buy and inconvenient to take. Powdered zinc (in capsules) is also good if you can't get liquid. Tablets are okay if that's all that is available, but they are relatively poorly absorbed—your body gets only a small percentage of the zinc in them.

Zinc

RDA: 15 mg

Recommended dose (general): 30 mg

Recommended dose (in trouble): 80–160 mg for a few weeks at a time, in manic crisis.

Maximum safe level: Unknown; one boy who consumed 12,000 mg (12 grams) of zinc overslept for four days, fell asleep frequently through the day, wrote in illegible scrawl, staggered when he walked. Completely recovered sixth day, no permanent harm.

Contraindications: Coma

DHA

The essential fatty acid DHA (which is called by its acronym to save us all from having to repeat "docosahexaenoic acid"), not to be confused with the hormone DHEA, is an omega-3 oil found in fish and seaweed. It is "essential" in several ways, including building the physical brain (as well as the retina) and developing brain function throughout life. Low blood levels of DHA predict low serotonin, and low levels of DHA have been linked to depression (and schizophrenia), among many other things. Lower DHA levels are associated with more severe symptoms of depression than levels that are still insufficient but not quite as low. That is, the lower your DHA level, the more severe your depression may be.

Americans have among the lowest DHA levels anywhere in the world, perhaps because we eat less seafood than many other cultures. Fortunately, we know simple ways to get more of it in our diets and have a choice of supplements as well. Studies have proven that DHA supplements can prevent, reverse, or slow the progression of the health problems linked to it, including depression.

The best source of DHA is cold-water fish like salmon, tuna, and sardines. Other fish also have DHA, but in lower concentrations. You can also

DHA

Recommended dose (in balance): 0–1,000 mg daily (3–4 fish oil capsules)

Recommended dose (in trouble): 800–1,250 mg daily (4–6 fish oil capsules)

Maximum safe level: 5,000 mg a day for several months could result in harmful effects, though there is no reason to use it at that level.

Contraindications: None. Some people complain of fishy odor and taste.

get it from seaweed, such as hijiki, nori, and kombu, if you're willing to experiment with what you can find at your health food store (or Asian grocery). Some chicken and eggs may contain DHA if the chickens are raised on special feed rich in DHA, so watch for labels touting this added benefit. According to the label on a dozen of these special eggs purchased at my local organic food store, there is 300 mg of DHA in two eggs, compared to 36 mg in two regular eggs. (The special eggs also had six times the normal amount of vitamin E.)

If you aren't getting enough DHA in your diet, supplements will do the job. Most are made from fish. If you are vegetarian or are concerned about concentration of toxins in fish oil, supplements made from algae are also available. Fish oils have EPA, a fatty acid that thins blood, so anyone taking blood-thinning medications of any kind should consult with their doctor before taking them. Pregnant women should always discuss supplements with their doctors.

DHA is very unstable, so use capsules that have vitamin E added to prevent rancidity. In addition, take 400 IU of vitamin E along with DHA to prevent oxidation in the body.

INTERVENTIONS—FOR TIMES OF TROUBLE ONLY

To rebalance yourself when you are in trouble, several amino acids and herbs have been proven to boost serotonin or otherwise reverse depression, and the best of those are covered below. These supplements are not generally intended for daily use over the long term and will yield their best results when used in addition to a proper diet. If you are seriously depressed, don't treat yourself; use this guide only with the help of a knowledgeable health-care professional.

INTERVENTION	DAILY DOSE
Amino Acids	
Tryptophan	500–9,000 mg
5-HTP (an alternative to tryptophan)	150 mg 3 times a day
Tyrosine	1.5–3 g
Phenylalanine	1.5–3 g (L-phenylalanine)
	500 mg (DL-phenylalanine) 3 times a day for one week, then once daily.
Minerals	
Cesium	100 mg once every 3 months, up to 400 mg every day (only if followed by physician)
Accessory Nutrients	
SAMe	400–1,600 mg
Herbs	
St. John's Wort	300 mg 3 times a day
Green Tea	2–4 cups a day
Ginseng	2–4 cups a day as tea; or
	100–1,250 mg in capsules; or
	300 mg/ml in liquid form.

Tryptophan

At one time, this amino acid was my stand-alone treatment for depression, as it was widely sold over the counter in drugstores and health food stores. I treated hundreds of people with tryptophan, and in the majority of depressed people I saw, it was the most successful way to reverse their blues.

And none of my patients ever had a significant side effect. But the FDA took it off the market in 1989 after one contaminated batch made 1,500 people seriously ill and killed 37 people (though the exact numbers vary depending on who is doing the counting). The FDA is concerned with product safety, and rightly so. But the problem was not with tryptophan—it was with the contaminant. The repercussions of one bad batch were tragic, but it is also a loss to no longer have this safe, effective, natural antidepressant readily available.

Tryptophan for Insomnia

Tryptophan is an excellent antidote to insomnia, increasing sleepiness and decreasing waking time. (When the insomnia is accompanied by depression, it's a "two birds/one stone" deal.) A rise in serotonin levels can make you feel sleepy, and in addition, serotonin may be depleted by sleep. Because tryptophan is made into serotonin by the body, it supports the former and counteracts the latter.

For insomnia, take tryptophan about twenty minutes before bedtime. Hypoglycemia can cause insomnia as well as depression, and if that's your situation, a high-protein snack to keep your blood sugar stable through the night is particularly beneficial.

Your body builds up a tolerance to tryptophan, so the sleep effect will wear off after a few nights. It isn't a knockout drug, it just relaxes you, putting you into a more mellow state so you can go to sleep naturally. You can't use it every night, but for an occasional bout of insomnia, it's very effective. The good news is that if you're taking it for depression, after a few days it will no longer make you sleepy.

Depressed people generally have low tryptophan levels, as well as low serotonin levels. Since the body uses tryptophan to make serotonin, taking tryptophan increases the rate at which serotonin is made and raises serotonin levels in the blood and brain. Insufficient tryptophan can block synthesis of serotonin.

Studies confirm the effectiveness of high doses of tryptophan in mild to moderate depression, usually within four weeks. Other studies have shown that low levels of dietary tryptophan can cause or exacerbate depression. Meals rich in carbohydrates have been shown to raise tryptophan and serotonin levels.

Tryptophan is an essential amino acid—we have to get it from external sources because our bodies do not manufacture it. Many protein foods are one or two percent tryptophan, so all of us get some in our diets. However, the doses that are effective in combating depression are generally larger than the amount most of us are likely to get through food; therefore, we must use supplements.

Currently, the only way to get tryptophan is with a prescription, and you will probably need to find an orthomolecular doctor to write it for you.

Tryptophan

Recommended dose (in trouble): 500–9,000 mg daily

Recommended dose (for insomnia): 500 mg–1.5 g daily

Maximum safe level: Unknown. Don't exceed 3 grams a day unless you are under a doctor's close supervision. Theoretically, if L-tryptophan raises serotonin too high, *serotonin syndrome* can result, characterized by confusion, fever, shivering, sweating, diarrhea, and muscle spasms, and, very rarely, death.

Contraindications: Don't drive or operate heavy machinery while you are taking tryptophan. Don't take it with an antidepressant drug without discussing it with your doctor first.

Some other ways to increase serotonin:

1. Eat foods rich in tryptophan, including milk, cottage cheese, poultry, eggs, red meats, soybeans, tofu, and nuts, especially almonds.
2. Get regular pleasant outdoor exercise.
3. Avoid addiction to antinutrient substances like caffeine, alcohol, white sugar, white flour, and white rice.

Your local pharmacy is unlikely to stock it, so you'll probably have to use a special compounding pharmacy to fill the prescription. (A compounding pharmacy is usually independent, though most do a national business via 800 numbers. (See the Resources section.) Perhaps it *should* be available only by prescription—we're using very high doses, like prescription drugs, so they should be used by people who know how to use them properly and who are being supervised by someone who can deal with possible (if unlikely) side effects of therapeutic dosage levels. It also ensures that you get pharmaceutical grade and that the FDA is watching it closely to be sure it is pure. Still, it should be more easily available—having it at most pharmacies would be a step in the right direction.

Prescription tryptophan is relatively expensive (not to mention relatively inconvenient). Most amino acids are costly, which is why I prefer vitamins whenever possible. Vitamins are generally less expensive, and they are also less likely to upset the body's metabolic balance than the more complex amino acids. Still, amino acids are quite safe, and no specific problems have been traced to taking amino acid supplements. And they have very real advantages: They are often stronger than vitamins, and they work more rapidly.

For example, sometimes I recommend niacin in place of tryptophan. Our bodies convert niacin into tryptophan (which is then made into serotonin). That's cost effective, and it is less of a hassle for my patients to get the supplement they need. But tryptophan would be a better choice if they needed something stronger. It would also work faster—you would feel its effects within twenty minutes.

The first time you take tryptophan, do so near bedtime, or at least not when you need to drive or operate machinery, in case it makes you sleepy (see "Tryptophan for Insomnia" on page 86). That's good advice anytime you're taking a new supplement.

5-HTP (5-Hydroxy-Tryptophan)

An alternative (and close cousin) to tryptophan that is currently available over the counter is 5-HTP (5-hydroxy-tryptophan). It is touted as safer and more effective than L-tryptophan.

5-HTP is one step closer in the biochemical chain to serotonin than tryptophan: The body actually makes tryptophan into 5-HTP, and then makes 5-HTP into serotonin. 5-HTP increases serotonin, along with endorphins and other neurotransmitters, all of which serve to combat depression. Studies show that 5-HTP's effectiveness is comparable to SSRIs (like Prozac) and tricyclic antidepressants (like Elavil). More 5-HTP actually becomes serotonin than the same dose of tryptophan would, so you need smaller doses of 5-HTP to get the same effect.

5-HTP may be safer than tryptophan, too, because it is derived from a plant, and so is not as vulnerable to contamination in the manufacturing process as is tryptophan, which is made with bacteria.

5-HTP

Recommended dose (in trouble): 150 mg 3 times a day (adults only)

Recommended dose (for insomnia): 200–300 mg at bedtime; repeat in an hour if you are still awake.

Contraindications: Do not take 5-HTP with psychiatric drugs without consulting your prescribing physician.

Is It All in Your Head?

Stoics in trouble frequently have many physical complaints or limitations—even those who have generally been physically active. They tend to develop a trick knee, or discover a heart condition, and often a cluster of much less specific ailments. You'd be amazed how many Stoics suffer from migraines. I think a physical ailment can be a good thing in that it gets many Stoics to a doctor, which might otherwise never happen. Typically, a Stoic doesn't see a doctor for regular checkups—that would require focusing on yourself and your own needs.

Of course these physical conditions may well need medical treatment. But often, just addressing the underlying depression will alleviate them, particularly the more nebulous complaints. It isn't that they are not "real," or that they are "all in your head," but rather that they result from the same biochemical imbalances that cause depression, and can be cleared up the same way. That requires treating the root cause of the depression, *not* just the symptoms, as is so often the case with therapy and prescription drugs. If a vitamin deficiency is upsetting your brain chemistry, you must reverse that deficiency. Something that just makes you *feel* better without actually getting any better will be short term at best, and certainly won't do anything about any auxiliary problems.

Tyrosine

Serotonin is widely known to be important in moods, and since so many of the pharmaceutical treatments center on this neurotransmitter, it is what we hear most about. But another leading theory of the mechanisms behind depression point to low levels of noradrenaline. The amino acid tyrosine is a precursor to adrenaline and noradrenaline as well as to dopamine and cortisol. All those neurotransmitters play key roles in regulating mood, and noradrenaline and dopamine in particular keep you alert, lively, attentive, motivated, energetic, and quick to react. Lack of tyrosine can lead to a deficiency in noradrenaline in the brain, and depression can result. Studies have shown that taking tyrosine supplements does raise noradrenaline levels and activity, and that can prevent or reverse depression.

Tyrosine also helps manage stress by raising adrenaline as well as dopamine, and studies show that tyrosine supplements can reduce symptoms of stress.

Many people do not seem to respond to this amino acid, but for those it works for, tyrosine is very effective. For sluggish depressions (not the classic Stoic "smiling depression"), tyrosine's link to the excitatory neurotransmitters adrenaline and noradrenaline may be particularly helpful (whereas sedating tryptophan may be more suited to agitated, over-excited depressions). Another way to gauge which amino acid might help you most—if trial-and-error is not for you—is to measure the amount of MHPG (3-methoxy-4-hydroxyphenolglycol, if you must know) in your urine. MHPG is the main product of the breakdown of noradrenaline. Low levels of MHPG suggest low levels of noradrenaline in the brain, making

---

Tyrosine

Recommended dose (in trouble): 1.5–3 g daily

Maximum safe level: Dosages of 10–12 g have been used without side effects. However, for depression do not use more than 1.5 g daily unsupervised, going up to 3–6 g only under a doctor's guidance.

Contraindications: Do not take tyrosine with MAOIs. If you are taking a prescription drug for depression, discuss its use with your doctor before you start taking tyrosine. Do not take it if you have active cancer.

noradrenaline-boosting tyrosine a good choice. People with normal levels of MHPG would probably be better served by tryptophan.

Tyrosine is also a precursor to thyroxin, the thyroid gland hormone, which is needed in appropriate levels to maintain a stable mood. The thyroid gland is involved with general metabolic function, including mood, and if it is underactive, depression is a common symptom.

If you have an underactive thyroid—something your doctor should routinely screen for (see "The Workup" on page 124 in Chapter 4: The Guardian for information about a complete checkup)—try taking 500 mg tyrosine three times a day. Some patients need up to twice that before they respond, and you can safely increase to that level if need be.

Vitamin C and pyridoxine (vitamin B6) help in absorption of tyrosine. Tyrosine can be made in the body from phenylalanine (see below).

You should take tyrosine with a high-carbohydrate meal, or on an empty stomach, to limit competition from other amino acids, especially tryptophan, and to allow maximum effectiveness.

Phenylalanine

This amino acid is a helpful antidepressant, though not as powerful as tryptophan. It is also quick to work—you'll feel the "upper" effects, mild as they are, within twenty minutes, and the full antidepressant effect within two days. This is not a good choice for severe depression (for which you should be under a doctor's care anyway), but for mild cases, 500 mg three times a day should help. (You can take up to double that amount safely until you discover what level works best for you.)

Like tyrosine, phenylalanine is involved with many neurotransmitters. That's because the body converts phenylalanine into tyrosine, which it then uses to make noradrenaline, adrenaline, and dopamine. These neurotransmitters promote alertness, elevate mood, increase stamina, and manage stress. Stress burns up noradrenaline, and getting sufficient phenylalanine allows your body to make more to keep up with the demand.

Furthermore, phenylalanine is made into the stimulant and antidepressant PEA, which is generally low in depression. (Chocolate is a rich source

> ## L-Phenylalanine
>
> **Recommended dose (in trouble):** 1.5–3 g daily. Immediate effect about twenty minutes after ingestion.
>
> **Maximum safe level:** Dosages up to 15 g can be tolerated well in some people, though some get headaches above 4 g. You should use no more than 1.5 g on your own, increasing to 1.5–6 g with the assistance of a health care provider.
>
> **Contraindications:** Don't take phenylalanine with MAO inhibitors. Don't take it if you are pregnant or nursing, or if you have anxiety attacks, diabetes, high blood pressure, psychosis, phenylketonuria (PKU), Wilson's disease, or skin cancer. This supplement is not appropriate for children.

of PEA, by the way.) Phenylalanine supplements increase PEA concentration in the brain.

This dual action makes phenylalanine the most often helpful of the amino acids covered here. Just about anyone with mild depression will feel an effect. But tougher cases seem to be more likely to respond to tyrosine or tryptophan. Results are very individual, so you may have to experiment a bit to find the one—or the combination—that's best for you.

When taking phenylalanine, begin with 500 mg a day, and increase gradually until you feel the effect—but not more than 3–4 g a day.

L-phenylalanine is the most common form, and the one recommended for stabilizing moods. Another form, DL-phenylalanine, is useful for chronic pain. It will work for depression, too, so if your brain chemistry imbalance comes along with some form of chronic pain (migraines, say, or arthritis, or PMS), look for the DL form. With the DL form, begin with a "loading dose" of 500 mg three times a day for one week, then downshift to one 500 mg dose a day for maintenance. The body stores up this form, so you don't need to keep taking the higher dose. You may need more for depression than for

> ## DL-Phenylalanine
>
> **Recommended dose (in trouble):** 500 mg daily 3 times a day for one week; then once daily.
>
> **Contraindications:** Don't take phenylalanine with MAO inhibitors. Don't take it if you are pregnant or nursing, or if you have anxiety attacks, diabetes, high blood pressure, psychosis, phenylketonuria (PKU), Wilson's disease, or active cancer. This supplement is not appropriate for children.

pain relief, and if that's the case, add in the L-form only (in addition to the DL)—up to a total of no more than 4 g all together. Unless you are also dealing with chronic pain, it is best to use L-phenylalanine only.

Cesium

I think of cesium as "ceasing" depression. This mineral was originally tested for its anticancer properties (though it is no longer readily available for shrinking tumors), and as a by-product, researchers noted that the cancer patients were more cheerful and more active on the cesium than before they took it. Though not widely used, I've found it to be helpful with several of my patients.

I've also had success with it myself. During a period of "holiday blues" and seasonal affective disorder (SAD), I read about the good results my mentor and colleague Dr. Carl C. Pfeiffer was having with cesium in de-

> ## Cesium
>
> **Recommended dose (in trouble):** 100 mg once every 3 months, up to 400 mg every day (only if under a doctor's guidance)
>
> **Contraindications:** Women of childbearing age should not take cesium, as we don't know enough about it.

pressive patients, many of whom had been unresponsive to any other treatment. I decided to try it on myself. Within twenty minutes of taking the first dose, I noticed I was physically more active. Within twenty-four hours, my melancholy was completely gone. I continued to feel good for about three months, which I attribute to that single dose of cesium. After that, I started using cesium with many of my patients who were depressed, with almost uniformly good results.

Cesium exists in nature, but it is a rare element. In the same family of alkali minerals as lithium, cesium does appear in the human bloodstream, albeit in minuscule quantities. Just one dose will raise blood levels to double what they were before the first dose, although even doubled the amount is vanishingly small. Your blood level of cesium goes down precipitously by four hours after a dose, and almost all of it is excreted within twenty-four hours. The trace amount left after that lingers in the body for a long time. Your body has only about seven parts per billion to begin with, so even a trace amount in addition is a huge increase. Levels will still be relatively high three months after you take that one dose!

Women of childbearing age should not take cesium. Because of its basic stimulant effect, cesium makes the occasional patient prone to nervousness complain of increased anxiety. But that's the only side effect I've seen, and it disappears within a day. Discontinuing it will also end that effect. Most people can take cesium without any ill effect.

The standard dose I use with my patients (men, and women past menopause) is 100 mg as a single dose when needed for depression. In mild cases, one dose is all that is necessary. Severe chronic cases may require up to 400 mg daily, but this should only be done under the supervision of a health care practitioner. Cesium is available over the counter.

SAMe

SAMe (s-adenosylmethionine), pronounced "sammy," lowers histamine, making it a very good antidepressant. It has been used in Europe, particularly in Italy, for more than twenty years. It is a natural product found throughout the body, but particularly in the brain. The body makes what it

> ## SAMe
>
> **Recommended dose (in trouble):** 400–1600 mg daily
>
> **Contraindications:** Consult with your doctor before using SAMe if you are already on antidepressants or if you have bipolar disorder. Do not take it with MAO inhibitors (or for four weeks after stopping them).

needs—but only in small amounts—from the amino acid methionine. That process goes awry in depression, however.

SAMe is necessary for the creation of the monoamine neurotransmitters, and it enhances the activity of serotonin, dopamine, and other brain chemicals. Low levels of SAMe have been associated with depression. SAMe supplements increase serotonin and dopamine and generally enhance neurotransmitter communication, thereby preventing or reversing depression. SAMe is also an antioxidant and provides protection against heavy metal poisoning (and the depression that is often an early sign of it).

Many studies have proven SAMe's antidepressant effects, and several have shown it to be at least as effective as some commonly prescribed antidepressant drugs—but without the side effects. It also starts working faster than prescription drugs. Even some patients who didn't respond to a variety of other antidepressant drugs improved on SAMe.

There is very little SAMe in food. Protein foods contain methionine, but eating protein does not significantly increase SAMe levels in the body. However, without sufficient protein, your body cannot make enough SAMe.

SAMe also needs plenty of pyridoxine (vitamin B6), folic acid, and cobalamin (vitamin B12) to do its work efficiently. Deficiencies of folic acid and vitamin B12 can lower SAMe levels in the brain (providing one possible explanation for why those deficiencies are associated with depression). Folic acid raises SAMe levels in the brain—one of the reasons it is good for Stoics.

SAMe levels generally decline with age, which may explain the higher rates of depression in older people.

Look for the 1, 4-dibutane sulfanate form of SAMe. It's much more stable (and less expensive) than any other form. It should be taken on an empty stomach, first thing in the morning, with the other supplements taken an hour later with breakfast. Most people have a rapid response to SAMe, with improvement within one or two days.

St. John's Wort (Hypericum)

The herb St. John's wort has been widely used in Europe for many years to treat mild to moderate depression. In Germany, where it is the most common treatment, doctors prescribe it twenty times more often than Prozac (the leading antidepressant in the United States). St. John's wort has enjoyed increasing popularity in this country over the last few years as a mild antidepressant and sedative.

There are at least ten chemicals in St. John's wort that act in relieving depression. Much of what is sold in the United States is standardized to .3 percent hypericin, but that is not the only important "active ingredient." It should be no surprise by now that the whole plant, rather than any single extract, is most powerful, and that the various chemicals play off one another to create full potency and maximum efficacy.

So it may not be surprising to know that no one mechanism of action explains exactly how St. John's wort works. St. John's wort acts as an SSRI, just the way Prozac and many other antidepressant drugs do. It is also a noradrenaline reuptake inhibitor, helping to keep levels of noradrenaline up (and preventing or reversing depression associated with low noradrenaline levels). In addition, it inhibits the secretion of cortisol, lifts dopamine levels, and enhances the activity of the naturally occurring tranquilizer GABA in the brain. Nothing else has been proven to work through so many key neurotransmitters and hormones at once.

Of all the "alternative" antidepressant treatments, St. John's wort has been the subject of the most, the largest, and the most rigorous studies. The many studies comparing St. John's wort and antidepressant drugs show, for the most part, basically equal effectiveness—and sometimes, superior results with the herb. St. John's wort has also been tested against a placebo to

St. John's Wort

Recommended dose (in trouble): 300 mg 3 times a day

Contraindications: Do not take St. John's wort with MAO inhibitors (or for four weeks after stopping them), coumidin, digoxin, protease inhibitors, and indinavir (for HIV), cyclosporine (for transplants), or photosensitizing drugs, including tetracycline. Do not take it while on medication following a transplant. Do not take it if you are pregnant or nursing. It can speed up the breakdown of (interfering with the effectiveness of) prescription medication including blood thinners, cholesterol-lowering medications, seizure medications, cancer medications, drugs used to fight HIV, drugs that prevent organ transplant rejection, and birth control pills.

prove it works biochemically (rather than just by suggestion). The exact numbers vary from study to study, but approximately 80 percent of patients find relief with St. John's wort.

St. John's wort is very well-tolerated, and it has far fewer and less intrusive side effects than prescription drugs. In fact, one study that found equal effectiveness of Prozac and St. John's wort noted that twice as many people dropped out of the Prozac group as did from the group taking the herb (though neither group knew what they were taking until the trial was over).

Few people taking St. John's wort have any side effects at all, but some do experience gastrointestinal upset, fatigue, restlessness, dizziness, dry mouth, or mild allergic reactions. One study showed that 11 percent of patients reported side effects from St. John's wort—compared to 36 percent of those taking prescription antidepressants. (And those numbers are higher than most studies of St. John's wort, most of which show only between 2 and 5 percent of patients having side effects.) Taking the herb with a meal, or starting with a less frequent dose to begin with, can help stop any gastrointestinal symptoms. Typical side effects from prescription drugs include anxiety, insomnia, sexual dysfunction, gastrointestinal upset, and dry mouth, often severe enough to make people stop treatment. Other benefits of St. John's wort are that it is not habit-forming, comes with no withdrawal effect, and is considerably less expensive than drug treatment.

Large doses of St. John's wort over an extended period of time, or an overdose, can make you photosensitive. At regular doses this should not be a problem, though it gives fair-skinned people or those with other photosensitivities another reason to limit exposure to bright sunlight. Anyone who becomes far more susceptible to sunburn should simply stop taking the herb.

St. John's wort comes in capsules, tablets, and tinctures, and can also be taken as a tea. Even though the .3 percent hypericin label isn't meaningful in and of itself, it is the best information we have that a product contains the most important chemicals from the plant, so I recommend looking for it before you buy. The most common dose is 300 mg three times a day.

Some people feel the side effects of St. John's wort immediately, and for some people it takes up to six weeks (just as with prescription antidepressants).

If you are taking a prescription antidepressant and want to switch to St. John's wort, your first step must be to discuss your options with your health care professional. Suddenly discontinuing antidepressant drugs can cause a severe rebound effect, pushing you even further into depression than you were before starting treatment. Your doctor can guide you in making a smooth transition, gradually cutting back on the drug over weeks while slowly building up the dose of the herb. Once you've been on the full dose of St. John's wort for a couple weeks, you can generally stop taking the prescription safely.

Green Tea

Green tea is the same plant as black tea, except that it isn't fermented. All tea may have health benefits, and green tea is stimulating.

A cup of green tea has 80 to 140 mg of polyphenols and 50 mg of caffeine (although you can buy decaffeinated green tea). You'd have to drink 2–3 cups to get enough polyphenols to make it likely you'll see an effect. You can also purchase capsules of green tea extract. Look for the ones standardized to 60 to 80 percent polyphenols.

Green Tea

Recommended dose (in trouble): 2–4 cups a day (under 300 mg caffeine)

Maximum safe level: 5 cups a day. More than that, or more than 300 mg caffeine a day, may cause restlessness, tremor, and elevated reflex excitability.

Contraindications: None

Ginseng

Ginseng is what is known as an adaptogen. Its chemical components have opposing effects on the body, and your body will draw from it what it needs at a particular time. Ginseng can, for example, raise or lower blood pressure, depending on your current circumstances.

Ginseng root contains several active ingredients, as well as B vitamins and minerals.

Ginseng helps your body cope with physical and emotional stress, including depression. It supports the adrenal glands, increasing energy and stamina and fighting fatigue. It also improves concentration and boosts the immune system. Ginseng is not given for a specific condition. It is a general, overall tonic. Various studies over the years have shown that ginseng beats placebo when it comes to lifting mood, making stress more manageable, reducing fatigue, and improving physical and intellectual performance—all with no side effects.

The most commonly used species of ginseng is Panax ginseng, also called Chinese, Korean, or Asian ginseng. Siberian ginseng, also known as eleuthero, provides similar benefits and is often cheaper. (Note that American ginseng does not necessarily work in the same ways.)

For fatigue associated with depression, both panax and Siberian ginseng are good choices. Ginseng acts as both a mild tranquilizer and a neurostimulant. It increases your sense of well-being and sharpens your mental functioning, but without any attendant nervousness. In fact, ginseng is calming and relaxing. It promotes tranquillity, yet at the same time it is invigorating and bracing (without the edge of caffeine). It isn't primarily an antidepressant; rather, it works as a nerve tonic for calming the agitation that can accompany depression. Though it is by no means weak, its effects are subtle and are very much dependent on the individual's nutritional status. A body accustomed to lots of junk food, beer, and coffee, for example, might not feel much effect.

Ginseng is not standardized, so it is difficult to know just what you're getting when you buy it. Studies in the 1970s tested fifty-four ginseng products and found 60 percent of them to be worthless (and 25 percent contained no ginseng whatsoever). We have no evidence that the situation has improved (or worsened) since then. Some specialized ginseng roots sell for fabulous amounts of money. While that is by no means necessary, you

---

Ginseng

Recommended dose (in trouble):
2–4 cups as tea; or
100–1,250 mg in capsules; or
300 mg/ml in liquid form, daily.

Maximum safe level: Unknown.

Contraindications: Don't take ginseng if you have anxiety, manic depression, heart palpitations, asthma, or emphysema. Do not use it during pregnancy. Do not use it at the same time as caffeine, ephedra, or other stimulants if you have high blood pressure or migraines or if you are sick.

should steer away from the cheapest products to ensure as best you can that you're getting the active ingredients you're after. Check labels for something approximating 13 percent ginsenosides or 0.8 percent eleutherosides.

Ginseng is available in capsules and can also be taken as a tea.

Using Natural and Prescription Treatments Together

After vitamin therapy has had time to take effect, many people can wean themselves off the prescription drugs that they had been using to control their moods—or at least reduce the doses. You'll probably see significant results within four to six weeks, but wait two or three months before making changes to your prescriptions.

The drugs given for depression (and other psychiatric drugs) are addictive, so you have to cut back gradually to avoid withdrawal or relapse. Your system can become so adjusted to taking the drugs that stopping the medication can cause the same problem you were taking it for in the first place. I see a lot of people who have gone on and off heavy duty medications impulsively, and these drugs are just too powerful for that. Your body's biochemistry needs time to readjust.

Work with a knowledgeable doctor to carefully decrease your doses, and you'll probably be able to get off medication all together—permanently. Slowly but surely must be your theme.

You may also find that good nutrition will make any drugs you're using work, or work better (not everyone responds to every prescription drug, just as not everyone responds to every vitamin). For example, if you're taking an SSRI but you lack tryptophan or niacin—crucial precursors to serotonin— there may well be no serotonin for the drugs to protect. So you'll benefit from the natural strategies in this chapter whether or not you take a prescription medication. Be sure to let your doctor know if you are doing both. Drugs and vitamins can work synergistically, so even if you don't intend to discontinue a prescription drug, a lower dose may well be appropriate.

Stoic Profile: Abraham Lincoln

If some mythical group of American Stoics asked me for help in choosing a poster boy, my nomination would be Abraham Lincoln. Of course I never met or counseled him, but reading the most penetrating biographies provides plenty of fodder for my hypothesis. But you don't have to dig that deep. The famous images of his boyhood—tirelessly splitting logs, studying diligently by candlelight, walking six miles to get to school, uncomplaining—encapsulate the hard work, perseverance, and determination that are typical of Stoics. His grim visage, as shown in just about every likeness of him, captures the physical expression of a Stoic nature. Even the language he used during the Gettysburg Address—sober, logical, calm, and filled with pathos—represents the strengths of a Stoic. Just the plain fact of a life spent in public service is a flag for the Stoic character type.

Stoics in trouble get depressed, and their depressions are often triggered by a loss. In Lincoln's case, loss has an unrelenting pattern of pathos in a life ended at age fifty-six by assassination. He lost his mother, Nancy Hanks, at age nine; his sister Sarah when he was eighteen; and his first true love, Anne Rutledge, when he was twenty-six. He lost his son Eddie when he was forty; his father when he was forty-one; and a second son, Willie, died when he was fifty-three, during the Civil War. Most experts trace his melancholy and moodiness—his bouts of depression, really—to the tragedy of losing his mother so young, a tragedy that was surely compounded by repetition.

Lincoln suffered a series of depressions throughout his life that on one or two occasions verged on madness. He was first thrown into the depths of depression—to the point where his friends had him under a form of suicide watch—by the death of the woman he

(continued)

Stoic Profile: Abraham Lincoln *(continued)*

described as the love of his life and had planned to marry, Ann Rutledge.

When nature put before him a repetition of the tragedy he had as a child (losing the woman he loved above all others), it proved to be too much for him. His depression was so profound at times that it is said he never dared carry a knife. Living as he did in the Time Before Prozac, he eventually overcame complete dysfunction in this case by going to stay with a good friend. But most of the time, he didn't react dramatically to the losses, and instead just tried to keep going on with his life like a good soldier and a true Stoic. Others, like Warriors, for example, might have lashed out angrily. But he maintained his kind nature. And his Stoic nature stood out when he advised a friend that "when feeling sad, work is a cure."

Even as a young boy, Lincoln existed for other people's approval. "All that I am or ever hope to be I owe to her," he said of his "angel mother." His stepmother described him as the best boy she ever saw, or ever expected to see—including her own son! He did all that was expected of him, and all that was asked. He was quiet, neat, consistent, reliable, and cheerful. He was never cross, and never complained.

As much as Lincoln loved his mother, and as well as he got on with his stepmother, he did not have anything favorable to say about his uneducated and barely literate father. Ever the Stoic, he kept his judgment to himself.

The danger for so many Stoics is that in keeping all the negatives inside yourself, you can become so anxious to please that you never express anger or disappointment. The Stoic's basic outlook—one that Lincoln seems to have shared—is that he is good if other people approve of him. Stoics need to learn they are good because they are good, not necessarily because of what others think about them.

Mind/Body and Lifestyle Changes

While good nutrition is usually enough to rebalance brain chemistry and stabilize mood, there are several psychological and emotional techniques and strategies that can also help. The first three I'll discuss here every Stoic should consider. After that, I'll go into avenues available to those interested in deeper exploration or in need of additional support. But before we get into that, I want to remind you that studying the types adjacent to—and opposite—yours on the pie chart (p. 28) can yield many helpful insights.

Beyond that, the first and most important step I've already mentioned: discovering your type and enlarging your perspective to include all the positives along with the negatives people tend to dwell on. For the Stoic, that means not only acknowledging your tendency toward depression when your brain chemistry is imbalanced but also claiming the loving, detail-oriented, nurturing, capable, giving, other-directed parts of yourself.

Step two, also already alluded to, is for those with flat curve hypoglycemia: Try to discover what "trap," if any, you're living in. Simple awareness that you are caught can be enough to help you find the exit. If not, it gives you a good starting place for what follows.

Step three is to develop in yourself some of the positive traits from the other types. We all have characteristics of more than one type, though one type will be predominant, as I've said. So start with what you already have—the "keepers" that complement the strengths of your overall type—and focus on building them up. You should also take a look to see what you can learn from the other types that don't necessarily come to you naturally.

Stoics are opposite Stars on the personality wheel, and those traits may be the ones most awkward for you—but also the ones offering the most insight about your natural tendencies. Stoics will also benefit from learning to call on some Warrior characteristics. Stoics could stand a bit of the Warrior's ability to look out for "number one," for example. (When you're "borrowing" another type, you don't have to worry about taking on the downsides as well because it is against your general nature. So you can learn to put yourself first without risking becoming too self-involved and losing sight of the good of the whole, the way Warriors sometimes do.) Taking another play from the Warrior handbook, Stoics could stand a dash of their impetuousness. Warriors are very spur-of-the-moment people. They know how to have fun.

Stoics should also look to the best of the Dreamer traits, which should be a more natural fit, as they are neighbors on the personality wheel. Like Warriors, Dreamers live in the present, and that's another attitude Stoics could make good use of. Stoics should also take particular note of the way Dreamers live the "don't sweat the small stuff—and it is all small stuff" credo. Dreamers (like Bob Marley) believe "everything's gonna be all right," and a little of this dream approach to life would be a tonic to a Stoic in trouble.

No doubt there will be times you feel uncomfortable as you try to assimilate characteristics from other types. Some of my patients say, "It's just not *me.*" Of course, if it was, they wouldn't be there in the first place. At some point everyone has to learn to be their better selves, but it isn't always easy. At first it doesn't come naturally. It's awkward. It's a part of the "no pain, no gain" cliché. But after you've walked the walk and talked the talk for long enough, it *is* you. You won't know how you ever got along before.

Hippocrates held that the way to treat disease is to provide its opposite: for a disease caused by sloth, prescribe activity; for a disease caused by overexertion, prescribe rest. Far be it from me to argue with ancient wisdom, particularly when it so accurately applies what must be done in reaping all the benefits of your personality type while avoiding the pitfalls.

Do the things you are least comfortable with first. Do the most work on the most problematic part of your personality. For example, if you are shy, work on building relationships. You don't have to try to love the limelight or transform into a gregarious extrovert. But you don't want to miss out on fulfilling relationships, and forming and maintaining relationships entail reaching out to others. The fact that you are shy means relationships are so important to you that they become scary. What would happen if you can't make a success of them? The only solution is to become more adept at relationships, even though that's hard. You won't be a consistently happy human being until you deal with the things that challenge you most. Go after the thing that frightens you most. Face your internal fears. Conquer them.

If you run from them, the knowledge of your failure will always bug you, and you'll never be the fully developed version of you. Stand and fight, and ultimately, you'll be happier and more confident.

To limber up the traits of other types that you admire, you can try some basic "exercises." The next time someone says or does something that irritates you, tell them. You can do it in a nice way, but do tell them. Turn down, politely—but firmly!—the next person who asks you to do something you really would rather not do. The next unexpectedly glorious day, weather-wise, take a vacation from your usual routine and do whatever pops into your mind. Longer term, study dance, theatre, extemporaneous speaking, or a similar subject to work on developing your expressive skills.

DIGGING DEEPER

For Stoics who want to delve further into their interior lives, there are a few basic areas to focus on. Stoic depression is often suppressed anger. Somehow, depression is seen as socially acceptable, while anger isn't. One of my colleagues is fond of saying that behind every depression is a resentment. Whatever the specific emotions, Stoics tend to bottle up their feelings. When they let these feelings fester, it contributes to depression. Developing the self-confidence to become more expressive and speak for themselves can interrupt that cycle.

Stoics often think they are valued for what they produce. They may even value themselves that way. They feel that to have worth, they have to be the best cooks, the best friends, the best writers, the best working parents, or the best go-to members of the team. But all people are important just because of who they are, not because of what they do.

Stoics need to take the message they hear at the start of every plane flight to heart: Put the oxygen mask on yourself before helping someone else. You need to feel good yourself, and good *about* yourself, in order to really give to others. (That's the part that ought to grab your attention if you are a true Stoic.) Stoics need to think of themselves first more often.

Stoics also tend to be overprogrammed and overcommitted. A dose of spontaneity—which is usually about pleasing yourself—is good medicine.

Try asking yourself, at least once in a while, "What do I want to do?" Then do it! Without guilt! Try it. You might like it.

Worry is a Stoic specialty—only Guardians do it better. Stoics tend to focus on a specialized worry, such as, "If I say what *I* want, and don't always do what everyone *else* wants, the sky will fall." Worry is a kind of anxiety. As you've already read, depression comes from pent-up emotions—which all start from worry. Say you feel Aunt Millie slighted you in conversation, and instead of saying something right there, you kept it to yourself—worried about what "people" would think and how Aunt Millie would react—and it keeps eating away at you. If you respected your own emotions more and had just spoken up, the whole thing could have been cleared up and probably instantly forgotten. Your way, it could go on to the point of ruining the entire relationship, and it will certainly poison your mind. Getting a handle on worry (see "What, Me Worry?" on page 110) is like vaccinating yourself against depression in the future.

Ninety-nine percent of the things we worry about never happen. The things that do happen are the things we'd never dream of. So, why worry? You really can't "Be Prepared," Boy Scout or no, because you never truly know what's going to happen. The best preparation, then, is tranquility, and a belief that everything will be all right. You simply can't worry about everything. For a Stoic, realizing you don't have to is a great relief.

TALK THERAPY

For Stoics, just the act of seeking help can be a step in the right direction because they are making their needs a priority. For Stoics interested enough in really "working" psychologically with a professional, three schools of talk therapy are especially helpful: insight, supportive, and expressive.

Insight psychotherapy is centered on self-understanding, especially our understanding of the origin, nature, and mechanisms of our attitudes and behavior. The Woody Allen ideal (therapist as broken record restating what the patient says and asking how he feels about it) fits into the insight school. Shrewd guidance from a practitioner of this art gives you the ability to observe yourself and develop ideas about how you are behaving and how you could behave better.

To really benefit from insight psychotherapy, you must be intelligent and sober. You have to look honestly and think analytically about your thoughts and feelings. You have to be ready to take stock and be willing to make changes. If you are convinced that you are free of problems, insight therapy won't do much for you. Insight therapy can be disturbing (at least occasionally, if you are doing it right), so you have to be willing and able to withstand that with a higher goal in mind. For Stoics who haven't always paid a lot of attention to themselves on their own, having another person, especially an authority figure, take an interest in their lives can in and of itself be a corrective emotional experience.

Supportive therapy is a technique of psychotherapy aiming at reinforcing patients' defenses and helping them suppress disturbing psychological material. It uses such measures as inspiration, reassurance, suggestion, persuasion, counseling, and reeducation. It avoids probing patients' potentially disturbing conflicts in depth.

Supportive therapy is generally for people in an acute state of grief or anxiety, where they can't (at the moment) think about how they got into their problems. If you seek therapy because you are unusually distraught after the death of your father, a supportive therapist will first give comfort—not start in with a question about why you hated your father. Supportive therapy gives you, literally, emotional support, rather than the "cold mirror" Freud thought was ideal. Whereas in insight therapy, the therapist's job is to be objective and non-intrusive, in supportive therapy, the idea is to be an active, friendly partisan, providing direction and concrete suggestions.

Expressive therapy—like primal therapy (involving banging and screaming at the top of your lungs) and Gestalt therapy—aims at acting out emotions. It isn't strictly intellectual, as with more traditional streams of therapy. For Stoics who tend toward suppressing emotion, working this way can be difficult at first but also incredibly freeing.

Most therapy is ideally a mixture of insight and supportive psychotherapy, though most therapists emphasize one or the other. So ask about the path the person you're thinking of working with is most likely to take, so you can be sure it is a good match for you.

What, Me Worry?

When you are worrying, no one can really talk to you. You are not open. Your mind is not free and clear—the state of mind you must be in to receive ideas and inspirations—when it is locked in worry overdrive. Try these techniques to tame worry in your life and free up all that space and energy.

- Focus more in the present as one good defense against worry, which is by definition about the past or future. Ask yourself if you are worrying about something which you can (or should) control—and if not: don't worry!

- Catch yourself when you are worrying—and change tracks. Visualize a tranquil, beautiful place like a sylvan lake or a lovely landscape or meadow. Or Las Vegas, for that matter, if it works for you. Or fix your mind on God, if you find strength in spirituality.

- Make worry "ego dystonic." Anyone who has a habit that's actually detrimental, like constant worrying, usually has that symptom because they value it for some reason. They feel it is helpful. For example, a Stoic might feel that worrying prepares them for every eventuality. Making it "ego dystonic," as the psychiatrists say, means realizing that the symptom in question is *not* in your own self-interest—learning to view the symptom as a negative, not a positive. To help you on your way: According to studies of the body's biochemistry, worry ages the body more rapidly than normal. Besides aging you, worry is also wasting your time. If you're preoccupied with it, you're not using your brain in the full sense.

- Discover the power of positive thinking. Whatever happens to you, assume there's something good in it. For example, if someone swerves in front of you, cutting you off on the freeway, assume it is to your benefit: a reminder to slow down, perhaps—maybe there's a speed trap around the bend!

- Check the mirror for a wrinkled forehead. Take note of how often it is there. Erase it.

The Guardian

4

To understand the Guardian type, think Woody Allen. He no doubt needs the Guardian traits of attention to detail, perfectionism, and perseverance to produce the kind of detailed movies he does. To make them independently, he surely needs the reliability, parsimoniousness, and workaholism that are additional Guardian hallmarks. Woody Allen's cosmopolitan, sophisticated intelligence is typical of the Guardian. Guardians are also stubborn and conscientious. And they like to control their world. I'd say writing, directing, and starring in your own work gives you about as much control as anyone ever gets!

Guardians are, literally, guarded, and on their guard. They are safety-conscious, and forever watchful for danger of all kinds. They are always vigilant, cautious, careful, and prudent. (Guardians everywhere were stocked up with water, batteries, canned goods, and cash well in advance of New Year's Eve 1999.) They are looking for security for themselves and their loved ones. (Guardians join the PTA to lead a crusade to improve the safety of the school's playground equipment.)

In service of this cause, Guardians are alert, observant, thorough, painstaking, and precise. This makes the Guardian stable, steadfast, dependable, responsible, dedicated, and trustworthy. Your accountant is probably a Guardian. Guardians also make good lifeguards. Guardians get to the airport two hours early and always read the safety brochure in the seat pocket in front of them. Come to think of it, they'd make good air traffic controllers, too.

Guardians had those plane tickets in hand months in advance, having carefully researched the best deals and most favorable routes. That's because Guardians are planners. They don't do "spontaneous." Guardians are very organized. They were the early adapters of the Palm Pilot, and before that the Filo-fax. Their desks are neat and organized, with a comprehensive filing system at the ready. Guardians make lists, fully fund their retirement accounts, buy insurance, and invest in precious metals.

Guardians are creatures of habit. They like routine. They keep regular hours and generally get the routine of living down to an exact science that would make a professional efficiency expert proud. They go to bed at the same time every night and get up at the same time every morning. They eat the same thing for breakfast every day. They pack the next day's lunch the night before. Guardians probably have a particular diet they are following, be it low-salt, nonfat, scrupulously vegetarian, or no sugar. And they no doubt have a well-thought-out rationale for every last thing they do.

To a Guardian, anything worth doing is worth doing well. Their quest for perfection makes Guardians capable, proficient, persistent, and productive. They are also particular, meticulous, and exacting. Guardians get things done—in their own lives and, in fact, in the wider world. Society's wheels could not keep turning without a lot of Guardians on the job.

Guardians are often fastidious neatniks. They believe in "a place for everything, and everything in its place." Guardians are also often packrats (a result of the collision between their drives to be thrifty and to always be prepared). They maintain prize collections, like wines, coins, ticket stubs, CDs, roses, or books, to give just a few examples. Scratch a librarian and there's a good chance you'll uncover a Guardian.

The ideal job for a Guardian would involve a predictable routine and ordered surroundings. Careful as they are with their money, money isn't what drives them in their choice of work. In any case, they are hard workers.

Guardians would be good with a long-term, complex research project, for example, whether in the science lab or historical archives. Wherever they work, when the boss announces that the deadline for the year's biggest project is being moved up two weeks, the Guardians are the ones who immediately set about redoing their schedule diagrams, working out the most efficient way to shave time off the process, keeping everything on time without cutting any corners.

Guardians are highly intelligent, rigorous thinkers, often with a mathematical or scientific bent. They are logical, rational, sensible, and authoritative. If they teach you something, or offer you advice, you can be sure it is well grounded. Guardians are staid, sober, solemn, level-headed, thoughtful, and strict.

Guardians live by strict principles and are highly moral and ethical. They are honest, truthful, and honorable. They are also aboveboard and direct. Guardians are as good as their word.

Guardians are faithful, loyal, and devoted life companions—once they have made a commitment to a love relationship or a friendship. (That commitment is sometimes hard to make, however—more on that in a minute.) They are earnest, sincere, and fervent. If you get involved with a Guardian, rest assured you've got someone you can count on, someone who has your best interests at heart. That is, when they are in balance.

The Guardians' downfall is that they can become too rigid. When they are out of balance, Guardians can have difficulty making a decision or commitment, as their detailed analyses of every last option can lead to paralyzing ambivalence. Guardians in trouble are not good at direct expression of their most powerful emotions because their potency feels like a loss of control. When imbalanced Guardians are angry or sad, they fight to control their situation but worry endlessly about all the ways they simply can't.

Therein lies the Guardians' Achilles' heel: anxiety that comes from doubt about their ability to perfectly protect themselves and others from the apparent randomness (uncontrollability) of life. In trouble, the Guardians' anxiety—really a defense against anxiety—shows up as obsessions (recurrent and intrusive thoughts, feelings, ideas, or sensations) and/or compulsions (conscious, standardized, recurring patterns of behavior, such as counting, checking, or avoiding). Psychiatrists call it obsessive-compulsive disorder (OCD), and current experts grant about 6 million Americans that label.

Most Guardians, of course, stop short of that, even when they are out of balance. In trouble, Guardians worry too much. Their brows are always wrinkled. They become extraordinarily stubborn. They get (and stay) tense. Their thriftiness turns to outright parsimony. Their perfectionism paralyzes them. They are hard to please and hypercritical. A Guardian in trouble can be a real stick in the mud—and/or a serious control freak. Guardians in trouble feel as if they carry the weight of the world on their shoulders. They feel as if everything is literally life or death.

But balanced and supported with good nutrition, Guardians are at their best. The promise is great. Balanced Guardians are adept, skillful, and accomplished, and they can be energetic and dynamic—really on the ball. They can be calm, cool and collected, poised, and self-possessed. They can be even-tempered, easygoing, and tranquil. Down to earth, Guardians in balance live with both feet firmly planted on the ground.

About 5 percent of people in trouble fall into the Guardian type. Men and women are diagnosed in approximately equal numbers with OCD. The

Type	General Traits	Beneficial Aspects	Harmful Aspects	Vulnerabilities
Guardians	Steady Reliable Other-directed Safety-conscious Attentive to detail Vigilant Conscientious Efficient Serious Fastidious	Are homebodies. Are creatures of habit. Like a routine. Save everything. Persevere. Can count Woody Allen as one of their own.	Worry too much. Get (and stay) tense. Are stubborn. Are parsimonious. Act as sticks-in-the-mud. Consider every option unceasingly. Are unable to make a decision. Carry the weight of the world on their shoulders. Become control freaks.	Guardians in trouble tend to get obsessive-compulsive as a defense against depression or anxiety.

Guardian Profile: Leonardo da Vinci

Guardians are often perfectionists. It is one of their greatest strengths, although also a potential weakness. Consider the case of the great painter and inventor Leonardo da Vinci, also a great Guardian—and a first-class perfectionist. He spent four years painting his masterpiece, the *Mona Lisa*. At the time, it was considered to be the highest achievement art could attain. Even today, despite 500 years of deterioration, it is the most important painting in the Louvre museum in Paris and is always mobbed with eager viewers. Yet Leonardo himself was not satisfied with it, declared it incomplete, and did not deliver it to the person who had commissioned it. How fortunate for the world that da Vinci took all the time he needed to capture that haunting face with the mystic smile. But for him, personally, it is a wonder he survived at all, spending so long on one small painting. Without a wealthy patron, the story would no doubt be much different.

Da Vinci, introspective like the typical Guardian he was, struggled to stay focused and not drift away on tangents in his own mind. He'd be working on a painting, then get diverted by some other thought, leading him to one of his other projects, like the invention of a flying machine. As he became older and more set in his ways, more deeply ingrained with Guardian habits, he produced less and less work, both because of his perfectionism and his distractibility from the immediate goal.

Also just like a Guardian in trouble, da Vinci had a difficult love life. Guardians may get stuck looking for the ideal person on whom to bestow their perfect love. Perfectionism may seem a lofty goal, but it isn't realistic, and that is especially true when it comes to interpersonal relationships. Da Vinci never married, nor are there any records of any long-term companion or, in fact, any sexual relationships at all.

Guardian profile, however, is more common in men than women. Guardians are often oldest children.

Brain Chemistry Markers

If you don't think you're maximizing the positive side of your type and feel trouble brewing, talk to your doctor about getting a blood test to check your levels of serotonin, adrenaline, nonadrenaline, GABA (gamma-aminobutyric acid), calcium, magnesium, and zinc. (You can also test GABA through a urine test, though it is less convenient.) These are all markers for the Guardian type. The results can help you know if you are a Guardian in trouble or on the edge—or if you're just experiencing the normal struggles that come along with being a Guardian. They'll also help you figure out whether the diet and daily supplements along with the mind/body exercises (later in chapter) are likely to provide all the support you need, or if you should investigate higher doses or additional interventions.

If you have any of the symptoms of hypoglycemia, you should probably

---

Normal Levels for Brain Chemistry Markers

Serotonin	55–260 ng/ml (nanograms per milliliter)
Adrenaline	less than 60 pcg/ml* (picograms per milliliter)
Noradrenaline	120–680 pcg/ml**
GABA	0–0.8 micromoles/100 ml (blood test)
	0–10 micromoles/collection (24-hour urine test)
Calcium	8.5–10.3 mg/dl (milligrams per deciliter)
Magnesium	1.3–2.1 meq/L (milliequivalent per liter)
Zinc	60–130 mcg/dl (micrograms per deciliter)
Copper	65–145 mcg/dl

* This is assuming you have your blood test sitting down. If you've been lying down for at least thirty minutes, normal levels are less than 50. If you've been standing at least thirty minutes, normal levels are less than 90.

** As above, this assumes a sitting down blood test. For lying down, the range is 110–410, and for standing the range is 125–700.

also get a five-hour glucose tolerance test to evaluate if you do, in fact, have low blood sugar. That's on top of the standard components of a workup that should be included in a thorough initial physical for every type of person (see "The Workup" on page 124). See also page 49 in Chapter 3 (The Stoic) for more on hypoglycemia.

SEROTONIN

Guardians in trouble often have low blood serotonin levels, reflecting a lot of crossover between obsession-compulsion and depression. A person with obsessive activities, like compulsive hand washing, will have the lowest serotonin. Obsessive thoughts also go along with low serotonin—but are not as severe.

ADRENALINE

Because the Guardian in trouble experiences anxiety, the cathecholamines, especially adrenaline, may be high.

NORADRENALINE

Noradrenaline, on the other hand, another catecholamine, may be low. Noradrenaline is an excitatory neurotransmitter. Concentrated in the inner brain, the seat of instinct, it stimulates the expansion of capillaries, allowing more blood flow to the brain. Thus it increases brain activity and alertness.

GABA

The calming neurotransmitter gamma-aminobutyric acid (GABA) may be inadequate in Guardians in trouble. The neurons in the brain are activated by excitatory amino acids and quieted by inhibitory amino acids. GABA is one of the most common (and most thoroughly studied) inhibitory amino acid neurotransmitters and is a major component of the central nervous system. Wherever neurons exist in the human body, GABA is there.

GABA blocks transmission of some nerve messages, helping control the cells from firing too much or too quickly. Without it, or without enough of it, the system simply burns out. It is literally overexcited. GABA has a soothing, calming effect. Low GABA levels can cause trouble, but even at normal levels you can run into trouble if your GABA receptors are inadequate.

The test for GABA levels is not commonly used, and your regular, mainstream physician may not be used to ordering it. Many naturopathic physicians are more conversant with the test, as are, of course, orthomolecular physicians. What it reveals is useful, so it is worth going to the trouble of seeking it out.

MINERAL LEVELS

Calcium, magnesium, and zinc may be low in the Guardian in trouble, while copper may be high.

Dietary Guidelines

Eating according to the plan laid out here will help you be the best Guardian you can be by maximizing your positive tendencies and minimizing those that hold you back. The supplements in the following sections play a role, too, of course, as do the mind/body exercises, but what you eat must provide the foundation before you can build upwards. If you are in trouble, or on the edge of it, you must be strict with your diet. Once you are in balance, you'll be able to take deviations in stride.

Guardians should follow a high-protein, limited-carbohydrate diet with frequent meals like the one laid out below to avoid or correct low blood sugar. They should also eliminate refined foods, especially white flour, white sugar, and white rice. They especially need to avoid stimulants like caffeine, which can contribute to nervousness.

Essential Foods	Danger Foods
Animal protein	Stimulants like caffeine and sugar; Refined carbohydrates (though natural sugars, as in fruit, are desirable).

The Guardian Diet

Following is an outline of how Guardians should eat. It is not meant to limit your caloric intake—nor is it counting fat grams, carbs, fiber, or any other thing that almost all other diets have you do. The primary purpose is, of course, to balance your particular brain chemistry. However, if you do stick to these general guidelines, and include a reasonable amount of physical activity in your life, you will also reap a range of physical benefits, not least of which is a stable, healthy weight.

Further below are lists of specific food choices that are helpful and harmful. If a food is not mentioned, it is basically neutral, and fine to include on the diet. For example, just about all vegetables are fine—it is just that the ones listed have particular benefits, and you should be sure to include at least some of them frequently and regularly.

- 5–7 small meals a day
- 5–7 3-ounce servings of lean animal protein (meat, dairy, eggs) at separate meals. Make at least one or two of them fish (but not shellfish), and not more than one of them red meat. Remember, 3 ounces is a *small* serving. Most 3-ounce pieces of meat would cover about three-quarters of the surface of your palm, though this depends on thickness. A 3-ounce serving is about the size of a deck of cards.
- 7–11 servings (½ c) of vegetables
- 2–3 servings of fruit
- 1 serving whole grains
- 1 serving nuts, seeds, and legumes (This is optional. If you don't have a serving of these, include a serving—but no more—of grain bran or germ, tomato, potato, bananas, or raisins in the appropriate category above.)

Basically, you're looking at five to seven small meals with "meat and two" as they say in the South—a serving of meat (or other protein) and two servings of vegetables, with less frequent servings of fruit and just a little grain.

FOOD	BEST CHOICES	GOOD CHOICES	AVOID
Animal protein (5–7 3-oz. servings)	fish herring salmon halibut poultry (chicken or dark meat turkey) beef milk cottage cheese	pork eggs dairy products (including cheese) tuna (canned) salami canned or frozen meat	shellfish organ meats raw meat
Vegetables (7–11 servings)	green vegetables (especially dark leafy vegetables, spinach, broccoli, and cabbage) avocado carrots eggplant	cauliflower alfalfa sprouts corn iceberg lettuce	canned or frozen vegetables with EDTA, preservatives, or added sugar
Fruit (2–3 servings)	pineapple plums	blueberries oranges peaches cherries apples	canned or frozen fruit packed in sugar or syrup
Grains (1 serving)	brown rice whole oats (including cooked oatmeal)	shredded wheat whole grain bread and cereal (fortified) whole grains	white flour white rice hydrogenated oils
Legumes, nuts, and seeds (1 serving, optional)	soybeans (and soy-protein products like tofu) lentils lima beans pinto beans walnuts peanuts pecans pistachios almonds sunflower seeds pumpkin seeds sesame seeds	navy beans garbanzo beans (chickpeas) cashews	canned beans, peas in sugar syrups sugar-coated nuts

FOOD	BEST CHOICES	GOOD CHOICES	AVOID
Sweeteners	maple syrup honey sugar cane juice		white sugar chocolate cocoa
Beverages	chamomile tea ginseng tea		caffeinated drinks (including coffee, sodas, and diet sodas)
Condiments and Seasonings	brewer's yeast		

Keep in mind these caveats:

• No more than one serving a day (each):
Red meat
Grains

• No more than one serving a day of *one* of the following:
Nuts
Seeds
Legumes
Bran and germ portion of grains
Tomatoes
Potatoes
Bananas
Grapes/raisins

Protein raises noradrenaline quickly, making it a good approach for Guardians low in that marker. Three ounces of fish or seafood (high in protein, low in fat, but including healthy fats) will raise noradrenaline within half an hour. And protein won't give you the crash that caffeine, which also raises noradrenaline, does. Animal protein is best for providing plenty of the amino acid tryptophan needed to raise serotonin.

Natural sugars like those in fruit are brain food for Guardians. PET (positron emission tomography) scans show that Guardians in trouble have increased brain activity in the frontal lobe, where thinking goes on, and in the brain stem (inner brain) where emotions register. Increased brain metabolic activity requires increased sugar. That can actually lead to low blood sugar overall unless you get enough of those natural sugars in your diet to fuel the process.

As with anyone with low blood sugar, exercise is very important to Guardians. For the Guardian in trouble, daily exercise is desirable. Since a Guardian in trouble is at risk of exercising compulsively (just like anything else they do), I generally suggest to my Guardian patients that they vary the exercise, maybe walking one day, tennis the next, swimming after that, and so on. (Only not golf; golf is a Guardian's dream—or nightmare: a slow-moving game with plenty of time to obsess over the last, and next, drive). Varying the exercise may make Guardians uneasy at first, as it goes against their desire for routine, but in addition to avoiding compulsiveness, it also helps Guardians learn to be more spontaneous.

The Workup

A complete, thorough, and detailed history, including pinpointing your eating habits, is the first step to determining how and why your brain chemistry is out of balance—and what you need to do to correct it. The next step is a complete, thorough, and detailed physical exam, including several lab tests. Many mainstream doctors do not regularly use some of the tests that are routine for orthomolecular doctors, so you will need to communicate clearly with your doctor to be sure you both agree on what is appropriate and necessary. Even if you are working with an orthomolecular or naturopathic doctor, you should be a full partner in your own health care. To that end, I'll briefly describe the tests I find most helpful, and why, so you will be prepared to be your own best advocate. Every type in trouble should most likely have:

(continued)

The Workup *(continued)*

Complete Blood Count. This should include a differential telling you how many blood cells there are, and how many of each type. This test costs just a few dollars, and measures several indicators:

- White blood cells. High levels indicate infection. The normal range is 4.0–10.5 10^{-3}/mm^{-3}.
- Red blood cells. Low levels—anemia—can cause fatigue, and may accompany depression. The normal range is 3.5–5.5 10^{-6}/mm^{-3}.
- Eosinophil cells. A high count can indicate allergic reactions; allergies, particularly food allergies, can cause depression. Above 5 percent eosinophils indicates an intolerance to something you're eating or otherwise being exposed to.
- Basophil cells. These cells store histamine, and their numbers rise as histamine levels rise. High histamine levels can cause depression. 0–1% basophils is considered normal, and 2–3% indicates that you probably have high histamine levels. You can use this result as a rough guide to histamine levels, so you can use it as an alternative to the histamine test. If you have an elevated basophil level, a histamine test is probably worth the extra hassle and expense.

Blood Test for Minerals.
- Zinc. Zinc is sedating and is crucial for cognition and intelligence. It works in tandem with copper—either a lack of zinc or an excess of copper will cause overstimulated nervousness, insomnia, and even, in the extreme case, paranoid psychosis.
- Copper. Copper is stimulating, and equally important to cognition and intelligence. It balances zinc.
- Magnesium. Magnesium is another "mental mineral," in that a lack can cause hypertension, agitation, nervousness, depression, and insomnia.

(continued)

The Workup *(continued)*

- Calcium. This mineral calms the nervous system, so you want to be sure you have sufficient levels if you are having mood problems.
- Phosphorus. Refined foods take a lot of other minerals out of your body, but phosphorus stays behind. If it is relatively high, especially if the level of other minerals is low, that means you're eating too much white sugar and white flour. (If you are simply not eating enough food to get the nutrition you need, you won't see the same contrast between high levels of phosphorus and low mineral levels.) Sodas contain a lot of phosphorus (remember, they used to be called "phosphates") and can raise your body's level of the mineral out of the healthy range.

Blood Test for Biochemical Markers. (Choose the markers relevant to your type as described in the chapter about each type.)

- Histamine. Treatment may differ depending on whether you have high or low histamine levels. Low histamine means a tendency toward mania, and high histamine toward depression. With low histamine, the mind is racing, and with high histamine, the mind feels slowed down or blank.
- Serotonin. Serotonin is our best indicator of biochemical depression (low serotonin) or mania (high serotonin).
- Adrenaline. Adrenaline gives a rough indication of levels of anxiety. High levels mean excess anxiety, generally speaking, although the actual test results are not as clear-cut and reliable as with the other markers.
- Cortisol. Cortisol is increased in depression and lowered in manic states.

Blood Test for Food Allergies. Food allergies can cause depression, and the test that looks for an antibody-antigen reaction for 150

(continued)

The Workup *(continued)*

different foods can help point out where you may have problems. It isn't always with the foods you might suspect.

Check for Anti-candida Antibodies. Because of all the junk food in our diets, and the widespread use of antibiotics, our bodies may experience an overgrowth of the candida yeast in the intestinal tract. At normal levels, the presence of candida yeast is normal, but when too much of it spreads throughout your body, out of control, that yeast can cause depression, manic behavior, or anxiety (among many other physical symptoms). As your body develops antibodies in self-defense, high levels of them show up in your blood.

The candida antibody test can be falsely negative, though, so I use it mostly to back up what I observe clinically, and I treat it according to the symptoms I see. The signs I look for include fatigue, itchy skin, acne, thrush, digestive symptoms (gas, bloating), fruity smelling breath and/or stools, white-coated tongue, menstrual difficulties, and headaches. Any or all of these symptoms could be attributed to other things (many are common signs of low blood sugar, too), but they are commonly associated with yeast overgrowth.

Thyroid. Depression is common among those with an underactive thyroid gland—the kind of depression that puts you in a kind of stupor, making you feel sluggish and unwilling to move. New research indicates that about 10 percent of American adults have an undiagnosed thyroid condition. Levels should be checked regularly.

Five-Hour Glucose Tolerance Test. If there's a reason to suspect hypoglycemia (including otherwise unexplained fatigue, headaches, muscle tension, stiffness, irritability, nervousness, cold hands, day-

(continued)

The Workup *(continued)*

time sleepiness, menstrual problems, stomach discomfort, and even cardiaclike symptoms), this test can confirm the diagnosis. I will confess, however, that the longer I'm in practice, and the more patients I see who have hypoglycemia (about 60–70 percent of my patients do), the less often I actually use this test. It is long, invasive, and relatively expensive, requiring six blood samples over five hours. And, if it does its job right, it will make people with hypoglycemia feel sick. So this is not a test to order lightly.

Now, in a patient with the symptoms of hypoglycemia who has a diet that is rich in white sugar and white flour, I'm rarely compelled to look further. And if that person starts to control their blood sugar, they can confirm it themselves. If it works, they are (were) hypoglycemic! Sometimes it is the patient who needs convincing that she really is hypoglycemic *and* that it is intimately connected with her moods. In that case, I might do the test for her benefit. Experiencing your body having an immediate reaction to a dose of sugar makes the connection powerful!

Natural Medicine Solutions

Guardians in balance can benefit from daily supplements; for those in trouble, heavier-duty interventions are called for. The following pages contain daily supplements and interventions for times of trouble that every Guardian should adhere to. For full details on the particular recommendations, see Chapter 3 : The Stoic.

DAILY SUPPLEMENTS

To support the diet and bolster the results, Guardians benefit from several vitamins taken daily. Where there are a range of doses, the lower levels are generally preventive—for general good health—while the higher levels are therapeutic (and useful if you are in trouble). The descriptions of each vitamin and mineral included here will help you make sure the supplement is right for you—no sense taking anything you don't need. The following section lays out the amino acids and herbs that are helpful to Guardians, particularly where a more proactive intervention is desirable. For more information on the specific nutrients, see the listings in Chapter 3: The Stoic.

Daily Supplements

Thiamine (vitamin B1): 50–100 mg*

Niacin (vitamin B3): 1–3 g*

Pyridoxine (vitamin B6): 100 mg

Balanced B complex: 50 or 100 mg of each B vitamin

Magnesium (chelated): 400 mg

Zinc: 0–30 mg

*Start on the lower end of that range if you are pretty well in balance, and gradually increase as necessary until you find the dose that is effective and that you tolerate well. If you are in trouble, you might want to start with a higher dose.

Thiamine (Vitamin B1)

For hypoglycemia or depression, 50–1,000 mg of vitamin B1 daily, taken with a meal, is very helpful.

Niacin (Vitamin B3)

Tryptophan in the body makes serotonin and niacin. The more niacin you take in, the more tryptophan you leave available to make serotonin. Niacin is best taken together with tryptophan (see Tryptophan on page 134) and a carbohydrate snack, at 1–3 g a day.

Thiamine (Vitamin B1)

RDA: 1.5 mg

Recommended Dose (in balance): 0–100 mg

Recommended Dose (in trouble): 100–500 mg twice daily, up to 500–1,000 mg twice daily orally but only under the guidance of a health-care professional.

50–100 mg IM (intramuscular injection)

Maximum safe level: Unknown. Not necessary to take more than 1–2 grams a day, which is known to be safe.

Contraindications: None for oral doses. Intramuscular injections of thiamine can cause anaphylactic reaction in very rare cases.

Niacin

RDA (men): 18 mg
     (women): 13 mg

Recommended Dose (in balance) for men: 100 mg
                                              for women: 60 mg

Recommended Dose (in trouble): 500–3,000 mg

Maximum safe level: Any dose that does not cause diarrhea, vomiting, or bowel upset is safe.

Contraindications: Take niacin cautiously if you are taking high-blood-pressure medication, as it could make your pressure go too low. Don't take if you have ulcers, gout, or active liver disease or a liver disorder. Since niacin raises blood sugar, diabetics should consult with their doctors about managing their insulin dose before taking niacin.

Pyridoxine (Vitamin B6)

Vitamin B6 is a necessary cofactor for converting tryptophan into serotonin and glutamine into GABA. Always balance doses of 200 mg or more with equal doses of B2 and 400 mg of magnesium.

Vitamin B6

RDA (men): 2 mg

(women): 1–6 mg

Recommended Dose (in balance): 10–100 mg

Recommended Dose (in trouble): 100–1,000 mg

Contraindications: If you're taking L-dopa (as for Parkinson's), check with a doctor before using vitamin B6 supplements.

B Complex

Brain function is compromised when B vitamins are low, and negative symptoms can occur when levels are still officially "normal." Find a B-complex supplement that provides 50–100 mg of each vitamin.

Zinc

Zinc is required for all metabolic functions. It is a part of the structure of insulin (and is in fact added to injectable insulin to prolong its action) and may influence the secretion of several other hormones. It acts as a sedative.

If you have low blood sugar and the cold hands and feet associated with poor circulation, these could be signs that you need zinc. Diabetics often lack zinc in their pancreases. Other signs of zinc deficiency include oily skin, hair loss, lack of appetite, apathy, and lethargy.

Up to 80 percent of zinc is removed in refining sugar and cereal grains. Frozen and canned vegetables are often treated with chelating agents (substances that bind to minerals and escort them out of the body) in order to extend shelf life, but they also remove much of the zinc and other minerals.

Alcohol flushes zinc and other minerals out of the body, which can cause deficiency.

A high-protein diet of meat, fish, seeds, and vegetables is rich in zinc. Herring, mushrooms, wheat germ, onions, maple syrup, meats, milk, and brewer's yeast are good sources. Whole grains, nuts, seeds, peas, and carrots provide adequate amounts, but fruits and refined foods contribute little or no zinc.

I recommend supplements of zinc sulfate or zinc oxide for Guardians.

Zinc

RDA: 15 mg

Recommended Dose (in balance): 30 mg

Recommended Dose (in trouble): 80–160 mg for a few weeks at a time.

Maximum safe level: Unknown; one boy who consumed 12,000 mg (12 grams) zinc, overslept for four days, fell asleep frequently through the day, wrote in illegible scrawl, staggered when he walked. Completely recovered by sixth day, no permanent harm.

Contraindications: Unknown.

Magnesium

The mineral magnesium is a natural calming agent for the nervous system. It also has a mild antidepressant effect and works as a sedative, encouraging sleep if taken at bedtime. It is also required for protein and carbohydrate metabolism.

Seafood and nuts provide a good amount of magnesium. Green vegetables can also be good sources. However, magnesium comes from the soil that vegetables are grown in, so keep in mind that if the soil itself is depleted of magnesium (as is often the case), so are the vegetables grown in it, no matter what kind they are. Processing wheat, sugar, and oil strips away most of the magnesium originally present, and the chelating agents used on frozen vegetables lowers their magnesium content as well. Soaking and boiling food (as in canning and cooking) cause further mineral loss (unless you also consume the liquid). Alcohol flushes magnesium and other minerals out of the body. Birth control pills decrease magnesium levels in the body, so women using them should be sure to get enough magnesium to compensate.

I recommend 400 mg of chelated magnesium a day. The chelated form is better absorbed than the inorganic magnesium salts (magnesium oxide, magnesium sulfate), allowing for more of a brain effect and less laxative action. If sleeplessness is a problem, take the full dose at bedtime. If anxiety or depression is the main problem, take half at breakfast and half at lunch.

Magnesium

RDA: 6 mg daily

Recommended Dose (general): 400 mg daily

Recommended Dose (in trouble): 600 mg daily

Maximum safe level: Unknown

Contraindications: Low blood pressure

INTERVENTIONS—FOR TIMES OF TROUBLE ONLY

While the vitamins and minerals above can be taken daily for an infinite amount of time, the following suggestions are better when you need to rebalance to get out of trouble. You most likely won't need them daily over the long term, once you get your diet under control.

See page 102 in Chapter 3 (The Stoic) about using natural and prescription treatments together. As for using more than one natural solution at a time: When it comes to the interventions, I recommend using a single product at a time so that you can more clearly tailor the dose to meet your needs. These natural solutions can all be safely mixed, but because they act synergistically with one another, each individual needs to experience how each substance serves them in order to understand how two or more taken to-

INTERVENTION	DAILY DOSE
Amino Acids	
Tryptophan	1,000–9,000 mg (3–9 g)
5-HTP (an alternative to tryptophan)	100 mg 3 times a day
Glutamine	500 mg 4 times a day
Accessory Nutrients	
GTF—glucose tolerance factor, the active form of the mineral chromium combined with niacin and glutamic acid	200–400 mcg
Herbs	
Kava	100–300 mg
Valerian	150–450 mg
Chamomile	1 cup tea 3–4 times a day
Passionflower	300–450 mg
St. John's wort	300 mg 3 times a day
Ginseng	2–4 cups a day as tea; or 100–1,250 mg in capsules; or 300 mg/ml in liquid form.

gether makes them feel or act. If you do decide to use them together, keep in mind that you will need lower doses of each one than if you were using it on its own.

Tryptophan

Though this is the single best nutrient treatment for Guardians in trouble, it is currently available only with a doctor's prescription in the United States, and then only from a few special compounding pharmacies (see the Resources Section). In most places outside the United States, tryptophan is still available without a prescription and at modest prices. For Guardians in trouble, the dose is 3,000–9,000 mg a day (3–9 g).

Tryptophan converts directly into serotonin, so it can correct the deficiency often seen in Guardians in trouble.

Obsessive-compulsive disorder (OCD) has been proven to respond to

Tryptophan

Recommended Dose (in trouble): 500–9,000 mg daily

Recommended Dose (for insomnia): 500–1,500 mg

Maximum safe level: Unknown. Don't exceed 3 grams a day unless you are under a doctor's close supervision. Theoretically, if L-tryptophan raises serotonin too high, *serotonin syndrome* can result, characterized by confusion, fever, shivering, sweating, diarrhea, muscle spasms, and, very rarely, death.

Contraindications: Don't drive or operate heavy machinery. Don't take with an antidepressant drug without discussing it with your doctor first.

treatment with the amino acid tryptophan. In one study, patients with OCD who did not improve with the prescription drug clomipramine did get better with tryptophan.

5-HTP (5-Hydroxy-Tryptophan)—see p. 89 for full description.
This form of tryptophan is available in the United States without a prescription. It may be as effective as L-tryptophan, but is new enough that

5-HTP

Recommended Dose (in trouble): 150 mg three times a day (adults only)

Recommended Dose (for insomnia): 200–300 mg at bedtime; repeat in an hour if you are still awake.

Contraindications: Do not take with psychiatric drugs without consulting your prescribing physician.

neither I nor my colleagues are experienced enough with it yet to know for sure. Take one or the other, but not both at the same time.

Take 100 mg three times a day on an empty stomach or with a high-carbohydrate snack to enhance movement into the brain. If taken with protein, it will have to compete against the other amino acids in the protein. Because it is excreted through the kidneys, there is a theoretical risk of kidney stones. Taking it with plenty of water will prevent this problem.

Glutamine

The amino acid glutamine is used to make GABA in the brain (with the help of vitamin B6). Take 500 mg four times a day to relieve anxiety.

L-Glutamine

Recommended Dose (in trouble): 500 mg four times a day

Maximum safe level: Unknown

Contraindications: None

Glucose Tolerance Factor (GTF)

I recommend GTF (the active form of the mineral chromium, combined with niacin and glutamic acid) for hypoglycemia since it dramatically helps normalize blood sugar. The dose is 200–400 mcg daily with breakfast. GTF is also present in brewer's yeast. You'll get a good dose in two tablespoons daily.

Glucose Tolerance Factor (GTF)

Recommended Dose (in trouble): 200–400 mcg daily

Maximum safe level: Unknown. No need to take more than 400 mcg, which is known to be safe.

Contraindications: None

Kava

Used for nervousness or insomnia, kava (sometimes called kava kava) induces calm feelings, reduces anxiety, and eases muscle tension. In small amounts, kava is stimulating, but larger amounts have a sedating effect. Kava promotes tranquility and cheerfulness while making you feel very laid back. Kava sharpens the mind and shuts down the chatter in your head. You'll become calm and reflective, as kava works to relieve fatigue and reduce stress.

The "active ingredients" in kava are the chemicals known as kavalactones, of which there are at least six. Most work as muscle relaxants. Kava is also a pain reliever, stronger than aspirin, and particularly effective against headaches. In addition, it can lower blood pressure.

The most reliable and safest way to take kava is in the liquid spray form,

---

Kava

Recommended dose: 1 to 3 sprays a day of liquid (60 mg of 30 percent kavalactones per spray); or in powder or capsules, 100 mg of 70 percent kavalactones daily; or 150–300 mg twice daily of the root extract (kavapyrones 50–240 mg); or as tea, one cup 2–3 times a day, and before bedtime; or as tincture, 30 drops with water 3 times a day; or as an infusion ½ cup twice daily.

Maximum safe level: Unknown.

Contraindications: Kava can exacerbate Parkinson's disease. Do not take it with alcohol; barbiturates, benzodiazepines, or any major tranquilizer, or any psychoactive agents; anticoagulants or antiplatelet agents (including aspirin); antipsychotics; drugs for treating Parkinson's disease; or drugs that depress the central nervous system. Do not take it if you are depressed because it can increase risk of suicide. Do not take before driving, at least until you are familiar with how kava affects you.

which provides a standardized dose. Spray the kava directly into the mouth, 1 to 3 times a day, each spray providing 60 mg of 30 percent kavalactones. If you take the capsules or powders, the dose for tension is 100 mg of 70 percent standardized kavalactones.

Valerian

Valerian is a remarkable brain sedative, from which I understand the tranquilizer Valium was derived. There are about 150 species of the herb, which are widely distributed in the temperate regions of the world. Discovered in ancient times, it was extolled by the physician Galen and was so highly esteemed during the Middle Ages it was named "All Heal." The active ingredient is a foul-smelling yellow-brown-green oil found in the root. In addition to valerian's antianxiety effect, it is a painkiller, a sleep aid, and useful for epileptics to prevent seizures. At the recommended dosages it quiets and soothes the brain. Frequent large doses can result in headaches, feelings of heaviness, and stupor.

Valerian

Recommended dose: 150–450 mg in capsules or as a tea; or tincture, ½ to 1 teaspoon one to several times a day; or plant juice, 1 tablespoon 3 times a day for adults.

Maximum safe level: 1,800 mg extract daily. 15 g root powder infusion.

Contraindications: None. Because of valerian's sedative effects, don't drive or operate heavy machinery. Do not combine it with alcohol and other sedatives. This herb is not recommended during pregnancy. Danger of habituation and addiction exists.

Chamomile

Chamomile is a mild sedative. Apigenin, the active substance in chamomile, acts, like Valium, on the benzodiazepine receptors in the brain, producing a calming antianxiety effect. Chamomile tea is widely available and can be drunk as desired as a relaxant, for anxiety or insomnia.

For an infusion for internal use, pour 1 cup boiling water (150 ml) over 3 g (about 3 teaspoons dry, or 1–4 ml liquid extract) of chamomile. Cover and let steep for 5–10 minutes. Drink a fresh cup 3–4 times a day.

Chamomile

Recommended dose: One cup tea 3–4 times a day.

Maximum safe level: Unknown.

Contraindications: If you are allergic to ragweed, chrysanthemums, and other daisies, you may want to avoid chamomile, which is in the same family. (You won't necessarily be sensitive to it, though, so it may be worth a try.) This herb is contraindicated in anyone with a known allergy to the compositae family (arnica, yarrow, feverfew, tansy, artemesia).

Passionflower

The herb passionflower is a sedative that I use primarily for insomnia, but it is also a mild antidote for anxiety. It stops the chattering of the brain that prevents sleep and causes restless anxiety. Dosage of the dry herb, or taken as a tea, is 4–8 grams; of the dry powdered extract (2.6 percent flavonoids), it is 300–450 mg.

St. John's Wort (Hypericum)—See p. 97 for full description.

This herb raises brain serotonin levels by blocking its reuptake. The dose is of 0.3 percent hypericin extract 300 mg three times a day.

Passionflower

Recommended dose: 4–8 g (dry herb, or taken as tea), extract standardized to 1.2 percent apigenin and .5 percent essential oils; 300–450 mg of the dry powdered extract (2.6 percent flavonoids)

Maximum safe level: Unknown

Contraindications: None

St. John's Wort

Recommended Dose (in trouble): 300 mg three times a day

Contraindications: Do not take with MAO inhibitors (or for four weeks after stopping them), coumidin, digoxin, protease inhibitors and indinavir (in HIV), cyclosporine (in cancer), or photosensitizing drugs, including tetracycline. Do not take while on drugs following a transplant. Not for pregnant or nursing women. Can speed up the breakdown of (interfering with the effectiveness of) prescription medication, including blood thinners, cholesterol-lowering medications, seizure medications, cancer medications, drugs used to fight HIV, drugs that prevent organ transplant rejection, and birth control pills.

Ginseng—See p. 100 for full description.

This herb is unique in that it acts as a stimulant, as if you'd had a cup of coffee, and as a relaxant, as if you'd taken a drink of alcohol—but without the negative effects of either. It also lowers blood sugar. Dosage is variable. You can chew the ginseng root, make a tea, or take capsules of ground-up ginseng. Massive overdoses of ginseng can cause ginseng abuse syndrome: hypertension, insomnia, hypertonia, and edema.

> ## Ginseng
>
>
> **Recommended Dose (in trouble):** Varies according to the source. Follow package label. See Chapter 3 : The Stoic for more information.
>
> **Maximum safe level:** Unknown
>
> **Contraindications:** Don't take if you have anxiety, manic depression, heart palpitations, asthma, or emphysema. Not for use during pregnancy. Do not use at the same time as caffeine, ephedra, or other stimulants if you have high blood pressure or migraines, or if you are sick.

Mind/Body and Lifestyle Changes

Guardians in equilibrium balance their cerebral, hesitant approach with gutsy, impulsive action when necessary. They can make use of a little of the Warrior's devil-may-care attitude. They, like Woody Allen, lighten up and round out their usually formal and serious outlook with glimpses of their sense of humor. As with all types, they should look for insights, particularly in the types next to—and opposite from—theirs on the pie chart (see p. 28).

Guardians are thinkers more than doers. Out of balance, they resist the doing because action makes them anxious. I believe anxiety is just suppressed energy—energy that is blocked because of conflicting feelings about directly expressing it. The more Guardians put aside their anxiety (and the obsessive-compulsive streak it can manifest as), the more actively engaged in life they become and the more freedom their keen intellects have to accomplish great things.

Organization, detail, ethics, and efficiency are part of what makes Guardians great. In balance, you'll be able to step out of the usual when it behooves you, returning always to your comfort zone, where you belong. If you find you are becoming more rigid than serves you well, good nutrition will end the lockdown for you. You may find it useful, or enlightening, to try on behavioral changes for size, too. I've listed many options below, and they may spark your own ideas. Don't make a habit of any of these things—you wouldn't want to submerge your Guardian self. But include a couple in your life each week if you want to limber up some of the traits you admire in other types (the Warrior in particular) but don't usually hit upon yourself.

Break your routine. Take a different route to the office. Change your morning routine (eat breakfast *before* you shower, get your news from the paper rather than the radio—or start your day with no news report—have herb tea instead of juice, or set your alarm half an hour earlier or later. Do whatever it takes to shake things up a bit and depart from the same old routine. It may be useful to change things every now and then, just to remind yourself you can.

Be spontaneous. If you want to stretch some usually squirreled away parts of your personality, try carving out some time and space in your life for experiences that aren't thoroughly planned in advance. Go out for dinner on a Tuesday night—never mind the chops defrosting in the fridge and your ten o'clock bedtime. Make no plans for one entire day. Go away for the weekend—without making any reservations ahead of time. Travel with a group with someone *else* making all the arrangements.

Escape perfectionism. Sometimes, other things are more important, and that is okay. Leave the dishes in the sink overnight. Turn in something you've worked over several times—whether or not you are fully convinced it is done down to the last detail. Stop fighting with your kids over keeping their rooms clean, and just close the door.

Do something you are afraid to do. Not something that will actually harm you, of course, but something you worry about nonetheless. Speak your mind to your boss or your significant other. Let your teenager borrow the car or stay out past curfew one night. Invest a small percentage of your savings in something speculative. Make up your mind within a few minutes of facing a new decision point. See how it feels, observe that you survive, and know that you can do such things when you need to.

Take a risk. Buy a stock (or, if you're already in the market, a stock with a high risk/reward ratio). Try a new sport. Go to a casino and gamble. Ask someone you don't know very well out to lunch. Make dinner without a recipe. See a movie you've never heard of. Pick up something you've never tasted the next time you go grocery shopping.

Do something frivolous and/or luxurious. Not everything has to be sober, serious, and worthwhile. Do something that makes you feel good only temporarily, with no proven long-term benefit. Get a massage or a manicure. Buy a red shirt that catches your eye, even though you don't really need another shirt and you already have a red one. Take a long bath. Look up a "joke of the day" on the Internet. Read the comics. The next time someone gives you money as a gift, don't automatically bank it—spend it, on yourself. "Waste" a little time, or money.

Let go. Clean out your attic/basement/garage. Put all those empty jars you've been saving in the recycling bin. Weed out some of your collections. Gather up unused stuff in your home to donate to charity. Force yourself to figure out what you really need and want, and then make time and space for it.

The idea is for Guardians to stay flexible. You don't have to become a Warrior—but there's no point in letting that part of you get totally rusted out either. Planning ahead is all well and good, and it's one of your best strengths. But you want to be able to change courses midstream when necessary, appropriate, or beneficial. Like anything else, it will require practice.

To Guardians I recommend techniques such as meditation and biofeedback, which induce relaxation and quiet the overactive, anxious brain. Because of their introspective nature, Guardians are naturals for insight psychotherapy, and it can be used to determine the underlying causes (and therefore best treatments) of anxiety and obsession-compulsion. Don't let therapy sessions themselves become a compulsion though! Agree with your therapist ahead of time that you will stop at the end of a certain period of time—say six months. Dream analysis and hypnosis can be similarly useful. These approaches may also illuminate lifestyle contributors. Guardians do need to be sure to stay focused and not obsess over or drift away on tangents in their psyche.

For a Guardian, the goal of therapy is to bring out their Lover aspect as well. Lovers in trouble get anxiety, too, but they are less shielded from their emotional selves, and they don't get paralyzed. Guardians should take note.

Take for example one woman I know, a Lover par excellence, who attended one of those crowded massive marches on Washington with her husband, a Guardian through and through. She ended up pulling him through the crowd to the fringes of the VIP section in front, where they had a great view of the stage. Her Guardian husband would never have even gotten it together to get to the march in the first place if left to his own devices, for all his concerns about the size of the crowd, the potential for personal injury, finding his way there, sticking with his wife in a sea of people, and on and on. He's grateful now that his wife "made" him go, and now counts that day as one of the high points in his life. This kind of balance between two people is terrific—but you can seek that kind of balance within yourself as well.

Case in Point

David said he came to see me for the same reason that brings most young men into a psychiatrist's office: heartbreak over the end of his relationship with his girlfriend. He and Michelle had been together seven years, since he was nineteen, and now that it was over (which wasn't his idea), he just couldn't seem to get over it—even three years later. "I'm depressed," he told me. "I can't fall asleep at night, and when I finally do, I wake up several times during the night, and then early in the morning."

As he talked more about what had happened in the relationship, it was soon clear David was a Guardian in trouble. He was a constant worrier. His main obsessive worry (among a sea of others) was that he would lose Michelle; it came in a hundred different variations. And of course, he had in fact lost her, which he took to mean he was right to worry.

(continued)

Case in Point *(continued)*

David certainly *looked* depressed, not to mention emaciated. It didn't take long to unearth problems beyond the end of his relationship, namely drug abuse and food compulsion. The two issues (which, it won't surprise you to learn, contributed to the downfall of his relationship) were intricately intertwined.

Before David hit adolescence, his mother, who had always struggled with her weight, brought home some "diet candy"— chewy, chocolate-flavored appetite suppressants. He'd lived long enough as the "fat kid," so he thought he'd try them too. Sure enough, they took away his appetite, and he began to lose weight. Encouraged by the results, he managed to get a prescription for a stronger appetite suppressant—an amphetamine. He thought it worked: He went from 5'2" and 165 pounds when he was fourteen to 5'11" and 155 pounds at eighteen.

By the time he was sixteen, he had become a full-fledged "speed freak." Besides that, he also no longer had a normal relationship with food. He couldn't relate to it. Eating scared him. He liked his thin self and hated the old fat self, and every bite of food that crossed his lips made him feel like he was back in that old self again. Over the years, his diet evolved to where he ate nothing until nighttime, because, he told me, as soon as he started eating, he couldn't stop. He'd gorge on candy, chocolate, pastries, and ice cream—then make himself throw up and use a laxative to avoid gaining weight.

All this fit right into the profile of a Guardian in trouble— obsessive-compulsive behaviors (especially around food, cigarettes, and drugs) and extreme efforts to control his environment. His nutritional state was obviously poor since he almost never ingested anything with nutritional value, so there was no surprise that his Guardian strengths were being overshadowed by the pitfalls.

(continued)

Case in Point *(continued)*

But at least he was staying thin. "I think I'm nice and slim," he told me. "Michelle always said I was skeletal, but I've got this spare tire!"

I had to agree with Michelle. David was down to 120 pounds. His cheeks were sunken, and his skin seemed loose on him. His joints and even his ribs were pronounced. The "spare tire" that concerned him was, in fact, the distended abdomen of a starvation victim.

David was an Ivy League graduate and had been in a Masters program when his food compulsion and drug use caught up with him, causing him to flunk his comprehensive finals. He dropped out and, with Michelle, moved across the country. For a couple of years he lived out in the country and supported himself by dabbling in drug distribution. He was never able to find regular work, and eventually he went on disability.

In the end, his food compulsion and drug abuse consumed so much of his time and energy that he had little left to give to his relationship with Michelle. She had moved out on him three years before we first met. He now seemingly lived for their sporadic meetings around town or at parties.

Lab testing revealed flat curve hypoglycemia (typical of Guardians in trouble), as well as a nutritional anemia with enlarged blood cells (megaloblastic, macrocytic anemia), which is caused by either a cobalamin (vitamin B12) or folic acid deficiency, or both, as opposed to small red blood cell anemia caused by a shortage of pyridoxine (vitamin B6) or copper or iron. David also had elevated levels of the lactic acid dehydrogenase, which can occur in deficiencies of vitamin B12 or folic acid, and a high eosinophil count, indicating allergies or a weakened immune system.

(continued)

Case in Point *(continued)*

To correct his anemia, I started David on a series of vitamin B12 shots, using the hydroxycobalamin form, which maintains an active blood level longer than the cyanocobalamin form. I prescribed 1,000 mcg twice a week, along with 1 mg of folic acid, for three months.

I also advised him to avoid white sugar, white flour, and white rice, and to get plenty of protein. This, of course, would be a huge change from his current destructive pattern. The thing that seemed to catch his attention was that eating well—especially eating protein—would actually flatten his stomach, though he was skeptical at first.

By our next session, however, he was already looking better, thanks to the diet and the exercise I recommended. His physique was improving, his muscles bulking up (not in the Schwarzenegger sense, but enough to make him look normal and reasonably healthy, rather than starved). He had successfully channeled his compulsivity to a careful adherence to the new diet and an exercise routine. Not that the compulsivity was desirable, but at least it was positively channeled—I knew when his body was well nourished he'd naturally relax a bit.

David did complain that the new diet was boring. I hear that from a lot of patients at first, but I find (as I told David) that as their taste buds rebound from an atrophied state caused by a nutrient-deficient diet, they learn to savor the subtle tastes of whole, natural foods. Almost everyone decides in the end that they prefer their new way of eating to the white sugar–laced plastic food they once lived on.

In David's case, as with many compulsive eaters, the other life lesson he learned was that food is no substitute for friends, love,

(continued)

Case in Point *(continued)*

and interesting work. With those deeper sources of nourishment in place, food goes back to being something you need to live, not something you live *for*. Whole, natural foods then become your own choice naturally.

Over the next few months, David realized how his bingeing and purging had enslaved him, and how he'd been numbing himself from a life that had become aimless. Soon he was off drugs, and even cut back drastically on smoking.

With all this in place, David's anemia was corrected, his hypoglycemia came under control, his eosinophilia disappeared, his depression lifted, and restorative sleep returned. He ultimately returned to school, completed a Ph.D., got off welfare, and formed a mutually fulfilling relationship with a new woman. He is now a successful Silicon Valley prospector—where I'm sure his drive, focus, and conscientious care, liberated from the downward spiral of his Guardian profile in trouble, serve him well.

5

The Warrior

Gloria learned to steal from her mom. When Gloria was a kid, her single mother didn't have much money. When they went shopping together and Gloria saw something expensive that she liked, her mother would switch the price tag with an inexpensive item of the same type before taking it to the cashier. It wasn't long before Gloria was doing the same thing. Eventually, she graduated to stealing through more direct methods.

All these years later, it's different. The things that she takes aren't expensive, and she could easily afford to pay for them. It's about the thrill, the excitement of getting away with it. When we met for the first time, Gloria explained all of this. She also complained that she felt depressed—enough to interfere with her work, sleep, and eating—drank excessively, and had a smoking habit that she just couldn't quit. She finally realized that she needed to get some help.

Not that Gloria was an eager patient, at least at first. Early on, she was always impatient and often rude, and once, she cursed me out in the middle of the waiting room when I ran late one day and kept her waiting. Those unpleasant behaviors dropped away as she progressed with her brain chemistry diet, but I'm mentioning it now because it was part of what tipped me off to her type: an aggressive, impulsive Warrior. Specifically—when she first came to me—a Warrior in trouble.

Lab tests revealed a borderline nutritional deficiency anemia, with the small and irregularly shaped red blood cells caused by iron or vitamin B6 deficiency (the two being indistinguishable). Her histamine was high and serotonin low, both of which are associated with depression. Her five-hour fasting glucose tolerance test showed her to be pre-diabetic. She had modestly elevated liver enzymes, indicating early liver damage (thanks to out-of-control blood sugar as well as alcohol abuse).

Gloria started to follow a high-protein, limited-carbohydrate diet focused on fresh whole foods and free of refined sugars and starches to stabilize her blood sugar and repair the liver. Red meat and green vegetables are rich sources of iron, which helped counter her anemia, and I prescribed daily iron supplements as well. I also gave her vitamin B6 to cover all the anemia bases. The B6, along with chelated magnesium, also helps raise serotonin levels in the brain. To lower her histamine levels, Gloria took the amino acid methionine and the mineral calcium lactate. I often use niacin to raise serotonin, but it also raises histamine, so instead, I added the amino acid tryptophan for the same effect.

Within two months, Gloria's blood serotonin had normalized, and so had her behavior. Her liver enzymes too were normal. There were no more episodes of shoplifting. Gloria didn't want to stop drinking altogether, but she cut down considerably and practiced "safer drinking"—always eating whenever she drank, and following each drink with a full glass of water. She kicked cigarettes completely. Now that Gloria's on an even keel, the spontaneous, persuasive, fun-loving, decisive aspects of her Warrior self shine through, while her more extreme tendencies are reined in.

The Warrior

Warriors are goal-oriented, driven, decisive, active, enthusiastic, and dedicated. They know how to have fun. They are risk takers. They are the Wall

Street traders, the bootstrap success stories, the Super Moms. Fittingly, you'll find a lot of Warriors in the military. Warriors are also commonly religious leaders, political crusaders, salespeople, entrepreneurs, and CEOs. Whatever the field, for Warriors it is never a nine-to-five gig, but a twenty-four-hour-a-day game. They are almost always bent on a mission. The mission isn't always about duty (that's more the domain of the Stoic), and it isn't always deadly serious. It *is* always something they get very excited about. The Warrior doesn't always want to accept the responsibility of leadership—though since they are persuasive and outer-directed, they are actually quite good at it, provided they keep their impulsive nature in check. They usually see themselves acting in the service of something larger than themselves. Warriors can be the ones up in the bleachers at every single home game, with their bodies painted in team colors and the fight song on their home answering machines. They can also be the stage parents bent on seeing their little ones in starring roles.

Warriors share with Lovers an "at-all-costs" approach to getting what they want, taking to heart Shakespeare's quote: "All's fair in love and war." Warriors in trouble can be Machiavellian, letting the ends—their ends—justify whatever means. But they usually know how to look out for number one without losing sight of the good of the whole. When warriors do get into trouble, it is usually because they are serving no cause but themselves.

Warriors live in the here and now. Unlike Guardians, who think at length about problems, Warriors respond quickly to any situation with action. They don't sweep it under the rug and try to forget it as a Stoic or Dreamer might. And Warriors are usually correct in their responses, provided their brain chemistry is in balance and they are not swept away by emotion. Warriors are doers rather than thinkers.

Warriors' essential quickness is both their main strength and weakness. They get a lot done, but they also make a lot of mistakes. Impulsive emotion, unchecked, is the Warrior's Achilles' heel. When Warriors' emotions get the better of them, it is usually rage being expressed. When out of control, the Warrior's impulsiveness causes behavioral problems.

When brain chemistry is out of balance it is as if the inner brain, the seat of emotions, becomes self-involved, determining its own actions and ignoring guidance from the outer brain's inhibitory center, which considers consequences. Whereas in balance, hasty impulses deemed too risky are kept in check. Acting on an angry impulse is self-destructive for all the types in trouble, but it is particularly an issue for the Warrior.

Contemporary psychiatry would label Warriors in trouble as having personality disorders. Under too much stress, Warriors pushed to the extreme are even capable of psychotic behavior. Perhaps because they deal directly and quickly with tensions, Warriors usually feel pretty good. It is rare for a Warrior to seek psychiatric help voluntarily.

Warriors often struggle with short attention spans. They get very enthusiastic about new projects but then become easily bored with them. Something else worthwhile comes up, and the previous project is left uncompleted. Warriors have a soldier's strength as they start out on something new, whether it's planting a garden, building a deck, or sculpting a sand castle at the beach. They accomplish a great deal as long as the project is fun.

Warriors in trouble—though not serious trouble—have brutal tempers and problems managing anger. Warriors in trouble are also hedonistic pleasure seekers who, like babies, want what they want when they want it. They live for today and don't worry about tomorrow. (This is why addiction is a common pitfall for Warriors in trouble.) They are very spur-of-the-moment. Advance planning is definitely not their thing. They rarely take blame for anything upon themselves but are quick to point the finger at someone else when trouble arises.

Warriors react with anger when they sense a threat to their security. Think of the person set off by a near-miss fender bender screaming at the other driver, *"What are you trying to do, kill me?!?!"* Warriors in trouble can also be bullies. They are by nature aggressive, but when their brain chemistry is out of balance, that aggression can cross the fine line from productive to destructive. Warriors in trouble sometimes run into criminal problems. (Psychiatry slaps a label of sociopathic or psychopathic on Warriors in serious trouble.)

Even when they are basically in balance, though, when jobs or relationships get too complicated or difficult, Warriors move on. Still, they are always honest with themselves and in their relationships. Warriors are modest, democratic, uninterested in showy status, and not possessive. They don't care much for convention or the opinions of others, and they are very tough on themselves. Warriors always strive to do the right thing. Men are more likely than women to be Warriors, in part because of cultural biases as to how men and women are encouraged to behave.

Warrior Profile: Moses

Looking at some of the most famous stories about Moses reveals a first-class Warrior.

When he returned with the first set of Ten Commandments and saw the Israelites making offerings to a golden calf, his anger and rage got the better of him, and he impetuously (just like a Warrior) threw down the two stone tablets and destroyed them. Then he acted—just like a Warrior—quickly, decisively, and directly, to destroy the false idol.

In fact, it was Moses' penchant for leaping before he looked that ultimately kept him from entering the Promised Land. Once when the people were complaining because they didn't have water in the desert, God told Moses to point at a particular rock with his staff and He would bring water out of the stone. Upset by the people's complaints, Moses shouted, "Here, you rebels!" and struck the rock. Sure enough, water gushed out. But because he diminished the miracle by yelling, and hitting the rock, rather than just pointing as instructed, God allowed Moses to see the Promised Land but forbade him to enter.

Moses was not swayed by the opinions of others. The biggest example is his refusal to stand for the status quo—slavery for his

(continued)

Warrior Profile: Moses *(continued)*

people—and the way he defied Pharaoh. In a more specific example (which also demonstrates his Warrior's tendency to want what you want, no matter what), he sent his first wife away and then married an Ethiopian woman from outside the tribe, despite the strong disapproval of his older sister and brother.

Moses was very persuasive, another Warrior hallmark. After all, he persuaded Pharaoh to give up his slaves. Further, he persuaded the Israelites to give up the only life they had ever known and follow him into the harsh, barren, sinister Sinai desert. He managed to convince a nation to trade its security for an unknown and uncertain freedom.

Moses also gives us a view of the Warrior at the extreme. As a young man—an adopted prince of ancient Egypt seemingly worlds away from his birth as a Hebrew slave—Moses once witnessed a taskmaster viciously beating a slave. With a quick glance to make sure no one was watching, Moses killed the Egyptian, then buried him in the sand. Here we have Moses as the worst of a Warrior. But that quick glance reveals he was not actually a Warrior in trouble acting with imbalanced brain chemistry. He didn't fly into an uncontrolled rage and kill impulsively. His outer, critical brain was right there with him, making sure he would get away with it.

This is a Warrior in balance. It is important to note that, like many a Warrior, Moses was acting in the interests of a higher cause here—fighting the injustice of slavery. (Later, as a prophet with a direct line to God, Moses is the epitome of the Warrior acting in the service of something much larger than himself.) His conscience needled him to right the terrible wrong (the budding of the Warrior's drive to do the right thing). He went on, obviously, to fight the battle in a more organized and awesome—but no less brutal—way. Just like a Warrior.

Type	General Traits	Beneficial Aspects	Harmful Aspects	Vulnerabilities
Warriors	Dedicated Fun-loving Charming Persuasive Passionate Spontaneous Calculating Decisive Direct Uninhibited	Take risks. Are on a mission. Are doers. Do the right thing. Seek pleasure. Are honest with them- selves and in relation- ships. Are tough on themselves. Can count Moses as one of their own.	Are extreme. Are impulsive. Have unrestrained anger. Have a hot temper. Are aggressive. Are quick to blame others. Believe the end justifies the means. Give no considera- tion to what others think. Are ruthless. Are self-involved. Are hedonistic. Are con artists.	Warriors in trouble run the risk of socio- pathic behavior and even violence.

Dietary Guidelines

The diet recommended here is designed to help Warriors be the best Warriors they can be, maximizing the positive aspects and minimizing the potential weak points. The supplements described later in the chapter play an important role, too, as do the mind/body strategies—but the diet is the crucial foundation. The further out of balance you are, the stricter you should be with your diet. As you regain good balance, you'll be able to handle changes more easily.

The key for Warriors is to get lots of fruits and vegetables and to moderate the amount of animal protein they take in. Many Warriors need a hypoglycemic diet—high in protein, low in carbohydrates, and devoid of refined sugars and starches. Animal protein is a natural for Warriors—most of them get plenty already. But they also tend to eat a lot of refined foods—white sugar, white flour, white rice, and all kinds of junk food—effectively overdosing on carbohydrates. Avoiding those sugars goes a long way toward balancing most Warriors. Most would do well, however, to also switch to non-animal proteins, especially beans, legumes, and whole grains, along with plenty of vegetables. For the Warrior in trouble, the foregoing is crucial. Warriors fully in balance will probably do fine if they eat a lot of meat, though they become less able to tolerate animal protein as they age. Warriors should avoid alcohol and caffeine, particularly if they are in trouble.

Essential Foods	Danger Foods
Fruits and vegetables	Excessive animal protein

The Warrior Diet

This diet is not meant to restrict your caloric intake (or your fat grams, or any other numerical indicator most diets rely on). Aimed primarily at providing a healthy brain chemistry, this isn't a weight loss plan. But this is a healthy diet, and when combined with a reasonable level of activity, you're likely to reach a stable, desirable weight—and be generally physically healthy as well.

- 5–7 small meals a day
- 3–4 3-oz. servings of animal protein (meat, fish, poultry, dairy, eggs). And remember, 3 oz. is a small serving about the size of a deck of cards. Standard containers of yogurt run 6–8 oz.—which would count as at least two servings here.
- 3–4 servings of non-animal protein (beans, legumes, nuts, seeds, and whole grains)
- 4–8 servings vegetables
- 3–6 servings fruit
- 2–4 servings whole grains (If you've chosen whole grains as a protein food, you would still be allowed 2 additional servings under this category.)

The majority of Warriors in trouble have hypoglycemia (all of them should be checked for it). They are particularly prone to the standard, "reactive" type (see Chapter 3: The Stoic, p. 49), which, in animal studies, has been correlated with hostile behavior. Low blood sugar levels have also been associated with a tendency toward aggression in both psychiatric patients and "normal" subjects. High-sugar intake alone has been linked to aggressive behavior, and decreasing sugar to calmer behavior. A study of institutionalized young offenders on a low-sugar, no-additive diet dramatically reduced antisocial behavior compared to placebo and compared to the time period before the diet was implemented. In a separate but similar study, investigators found that the worse the original behavior had been, the more significant the change observed was.

Hypoglycemia usually calls for a high-protein, limited-carbohydrate diet that avoids refined sugars and simple starches. That's just what most Warriors do naturally. They tend to be big meat eaters, and all that protein helps them sustain their strength and energy as if for combat. But protein, especially meat, can overstimulate sex hormone systems and thus spur aggressive behavior.

Furthermore, as we age, our metabolism slows and our bodies are less able to handle rich foods. The average adults needs about 25 grams of protein a day to stay in balance, maintain muscle mass, and replace hormones, enzymes, and antibodies as needed. The remainder of a high-protein diet—with 75 to 250 grams of protein daily—is burnt for energy or stored as fat. As we get older we need to eat less (and somehow thwart our modern sedentary lifestyle) if we want to avoid that conversion to fat, maintain a stable weight, and avoid the increased risk of a variety of diseases that comes along for that ride. So Warriors on a diet rich in meat may want to cut down on animal protein and other rich food as they get older. Substituting vegetarian fare—beans, brown rice, potatoes, seeds and nuts, grains, fruits and vegetables—can still provide all the protein you need for stable blood sugar levels *and* help prevent illness and even early death from cancer, heart disease, and other conditions.

Warriors might benefit from simply drinking orange juice. Orange juice

FOOD	BEST CHOICES	AVOID
Animal protein (3–4 servings)	pork beef beef liver lamb liver red meat turkey chicken chicken liver salmon tuna herring milk cottage cheese eggs (and egg yolk)	shellfish
Non-animal protein (3–4 servings)	soy protein (including tofu) Legumes: lentils lima beans navy beans soybeans garbanzo beans Nuts: almonds cashews peanuts (peanut butter) pecans walnuts Seeds: pumpkin seeds sesame seeds sunflower seeds	
Vegetables (4–8 servings)	alfalfa sprouts avocado broccoli (in fact, green vegetables generally) Brussels sprouts cabbage carrots cauliflower collards (in fact, leafy greens generally)	

FOOD	BEST CHOICES	AVOID
	eggplant mustard greens onions parsley peas peppers (especially 　red pepper) potatoes pumpkins spinach sweet potatoes swiss chard tomatoes winter squash	
Fruit (3–6 servings)	apricots bananas berries blueberries cantaloupe cherries citrus fruits guava kiwi mangoes melons oranges papaya peaches pineapples plums strawberries	dried fruit
Whole Grains (2–4 servings)	brown rice shredded wheat cereal whole wheat products bran wheat germ rice polish enriched cereal fortified bread	white flour white rice
Sweeteners	maple syrup	white sugar chocolate cocoa

FOOD	BEST CHOICES	AVOID

Beverages	green tea
	orange juice
		alcohol
		caffeinated drinks
		(including coffee,
		  sodas, and diet
		  sodas)

Condiments and Seasonings	butter cream brewer's yeast	

The Way You Eat Is a Crime

When Warriors' brain chemistry is out of balance, they are at risk for criminality. The penchant for alcohol abuse makes it worse (nearly one in two criminal acts resulting in a prison sentence is committed under the influence of alcohol). Other antinutrients, like caffeine and drugs, also exacerbate the problem. Another culprit: a diet high in refined sugar, paradoxically leading to low blood sugar levels, has been connected to violent aggressive behavior. Low blood sugar reflects a weakened biochemical terrain in the brain, allowing misfiring of brain circuitry, including unchecked aggressive impulses. A diet like that is also more than likely vitamin deficient, especially in the B vitamins, which are largely removed from foods where they naturally occur in the refining process. The B vitamins, particularly thiamine (vitamin B1), niacin (vitamin B3), cobalamin (vitamin B12), and pyridoxine (vitamin B6) have dramatic effects on the brain. Finally, low blood sugar and vitamin deficiency depress immune function, leaving the body open to the negative effects of cerebral allergies. A food allergen causes an upset state of mind, fertile ground for bad behavior.

provides the folic acid, thiamine, and vitamin C that have all been proven to be deficient in delinquents. A study of institutionalized young offenders revealed that when orange juice consumption was boosted, antisocial acts decreased.

A junk food diet has been proven to cause impulsivity, irritability, aggression, sensitivity to criticism, and hair-trigger tempers—all the signs of a Warrior in trouble. I don't know of any studies comparing that to a healthy diet, but a study providing a wide spectrum of nutrients via supplements improved behaviors of that kind.

Brain Chemistry Markers

If you recognize yourself in this type and feel yourself getting into trouble, talk to your doctor about getting your levels of serotonin, adrenaline, noradrenaline, copper, zinc, histamine, testosterone, and (for women) estrogen tested. These are markers for the Warrior, and the results can help you confirm your primary type, clarify if you are in trouble, and pinpoint the solutions that are most likely to work for you. (For details about these tests, see "The Workup" on page 124, in Chapter 4: The Guardian.) And for more details on the markers themselves, see Chapter 3: The Stoic.

SEROTONIN

The primary brain chemical marker for the Warrior in trouble is serotonin, which is often low, but not always.

ADRENALINE

Warriors typically have high adrenaline levels. High adrenaline levels have been implicated in impulse disorders and are associated with states of rage.

NORADRENALINE

Low noradrenaline has also been tied to impulse disorders and is commonly found in Warriors, particularly Warriors in trouble.

Normal Levels for Brain Chemistry Markers

Serotonin	55–260 ng/ml (nanograms per milliliter)
Adrenaline	less than 60 pcg/ml (picograms per milliliter)*
Noradrenaline	120–680 pcg/ml**
Copper	65–155 mcg/dl (each lab has its own range, and whatever report you get will provide a "normal" range)
Zinc	60–130 mcg/dl (micrograms per deciliter)
Histamine	9–141 ng/ml

* This is assuming you have your blood test sitting down. If you've been lying down for at least thirty minutes, normal levels are less than 50. If you've been standing at least thirty minutes, normal levels are less than 90.

** As above, this assumes a sitting down blood test. For lying down, the range is 110–410, and for standing the range is 125–700.

COPPER

High copper is also associated with states of rage and is another sign of the Warrior. It has also been related to criminal behavior. Several studies of juvenile delinquents reveal elevated copper, and in comparisons of violent and non-violent men, the violent ones had higher copper levels.

ZINC

Zinc is often low in the Warrior, and the copper to zinc ratio is often skewed in favor of copper.

HISTAMINE

I always check the blood histamine too, since either extreme—high histamine depression or low histamine excitement—can occur with the Warrior in trouble.

TESTOSTERONE

Warriors may have high levels of the male sex hormone testosterone, which increases aggression. (The female sex hormones diminish it.) It can also amplify anger and rage and encourage impulsive behavior.

ESTROGEN

The female sex hormone estrogen diminishes aggression, and low levels may be found in Warriors.

Natural Medicine Solutions

DAILY SUPPLEMENTS

When the Warrior gets in trouble, it's usually from the inner motor action/emotional brain slipping out of the control of the outer thinking/inhibitory brain. Solutions therefore focus on the care and feeding of the thinking brain's chemistry. Daily supplements maintain good chemistry and prevent imbalance; the Interventions that follow can restore balance to the Warrior in trouble.

Daily Supplements

Vitamin A: 25,000 IU five days a week

Vitamin C: 250 mg–10 g

Pyridoxine (Vitamin B6): 5–100 mg*

Cobalamin (Vitamin B12): 1,000 mcg orally; 1,000 mcgm/ml
   (1 ml) injected every three to four days—only "in trouble"

Thiamine (vitamin B1): 50–500 mg twice a day*

Niacin (vitamin B3): 100 mg–3 g*

* Start on the lower end of that range if you are pretty well in balance, and gradually increase as necessary until you find the dose that is effective and that you tolerate well. If you are in trouble, you might want to start with a higher dose.

The supplements described here support the diet and sometimes boost its effects. The vitamins and minerals we begin with are appropriate for daily use; the amino acids, accessory nutrients, and herbs that follow are most often used when you are out of balance, and only until balance is restored. Where there are a range of dosages, generally the lower doses are meant for prevention and maintenance, while the upper end would be for the type in trouble. Start at the low end and slowly work up if necessary until you find the level that is effective for you. Take only as much as you need.

Niacin (Vitamin B3)

The most commonly helpful nutrient for the outer, thinking brain is the B vitamin niacin.

Niacin raises brain serotonin. Niacin is made in the body from the amino acid tryptophan. Since only about 1.5 percent of tryptophan is converted into niacin, our brains need additional sources from our diets. For most of us, even under stress, 100 mg daily as part of a high potency B-complex supplement should do the trick. Three grams a day is a reasonable therapeutic dose for bringing Warriors back into balance. Flooding the brain chemistry with niacin in that way causes less tryptophan to be converted into niacin—so 17 percent more is made into serotonin. For Warriors in serious trouble, niacin can be used in much higher doses (1–20 g a day) for an anti-psychotic effect (only under a doctor's care for 5 or more grams a day). Niacin is often helpful in clearing psychotic thinking and improving rational, cognitive thinking. In an animal study published in *Nature,* niacin had "anti-conflict, anti-aggressive, muscle relaxant and hypnotic actions with effectiveness similar to that of minor tranquilizers."

If you take in more niacin than your body needs and can handle, nausea, vomiting, diarrhea, and digestive disturbances may result. Should that happen, simply lower your dose to one gram below the level that caused the problem.

In doses of 100 mg or less, most doctors prescribe flushness niacinamide, which I never prescribed in doses of more than 1.5 g daily. At the higher dosage levels, I prefer niacin—and recommend learning to live with the flush (see page 71). For those who cannot tolerate the flush, buffered

Niacin

RDA (men): 18 mg

(women): 13 mg

Recommended Dose (general) for men: 100 mg

for women: 60 mg

Recommended Dose (in trouble): 500–3,000 mg

Maximum safe level: Any dose that does not cause diarrhea, vomiting, or bowel upset is safe.

Contraindications: Do not take niacin if you are taking high blood pressure medication, as it could make your pressure go too low. Don't take if you have ulcers, gout, or active liver disease or a liver disorder. Since niacin raises blood sugar, diabetics should consult with their doctors about managing their insulin dose before taking niacin.

niacin can reduce or eliminate it. Still, I recommend no more than 3 g daily of the flushless form (and would be happier if you stuck with 1.5 g), and you should have your liver chemistries checked regularly.

Even at high doses, regular niacin is safe. Extrapolating from a study in dogs, it would take about three-quarters of a pound of niacin to be fatal to an average-size adult human, and vomiting would occur long before one could consume enough to do serious harm.

The Nicotine Connection

Niacin is also called nicotinic acid, and if you think of it by that name, you won't be surprised to learn of its relationship to nicotine. Niacin can actually be made in our bodies from nicotine. This is one possible explanation for why nervous or upset people smoke—to get a dose of soothing, calming niacin.

Vitamin C

Vitamin C is calming and good for keeping Warrior brain chemistry in balance. But the research focuses on reversing negative states. My view is: If vitamin C can do all that at the extremes, how much more powerful must it be when you are strong to begin with!

Vitamin C supplements can suppress violent or aggressive behavior. In one animal study, for example, mice fought less with intruders when they were on vitamin C, and the higher the dose, the more dramatic the result. Vitamin C is an antipsychotic with the ability to make prescription antipsychotic drugs more effective. The study of juvenile delinquents drinking orange juice that I mentioned in the diet section above underlines the positive effects of increased vitamin C in the diet. Supplements work as well.

At doses of 1–2 g an hour, vitamin C also lowers elevated adrenaline.

Vitamin C is also crucial for counteracting the cerebral allergies that have been linked, in the extreme, to psychopathic behavior. Cerebral allergy is a brain chemistry allergic reaction, usually to a common food to which the sufferer is both allergic and addicted. Vitamin C in large doses has an anti-histamine effect. It also counters stress, and stress increases histamine, so it is double-acting. Vitamin C doses above 250 mg are sufficient to reduce blood histamine to a minimum. (It also works the other way around: High blood histamine levels mean low blood vitamin C.)

The recommended dose varies from 250 mg to 30 g a day (the later being only for cases of extreme tension). For general anxiety, use three to ten

---

Vitamin C

RDA: 45 mg

Recommended Dose (general): 1,000–3,000 mg

Recommended Dose (in trouble): 1,000–30,000 mg; use mineral ascorbate to buffer the ascorbic acid and avoid distention

Maximum safe level: Unknown

grams a day. If the anxiety is of psychotic proportions, higher doses of vitamin C may be needed. For example, one of my Warrior patient's brain chemistry was so out of whack that she believed passersby could read her mind. She was afraid to go out in public for fear of being "seen through." Thirty grams daily of vitamin C allowed her to rest assured that she was keeping her thoughts to herself.

Thiamine (Vitamin B1)

The B vitamin thiamine is especially important for Warriors who use stimulants, whether it's caffeine, drugs, or even thyroid hormone. Stimulants require thiamine for their metabolism yet are not sufficient sources of the vital nutrient. Following a fresh, all-natural foods diet and skipping stimulants altogether would be the best way to avoid thiamine deficiency. But until you get there, vitamin supplements are the best compromise.

I recommend 50–500 mg twice daily. There are no side effects even with high doses of thiamine taken orally. If oral absorption is inhibited, as it sometimes is with alcohol abuse, an intramuscular injection (50 mg) works well. The injection does cause a mild sting at the injection site.

Thiamine (Vitamin B1)

RDA: 1.5 mg

Recommended Dose (general): 0–100 mg

Recommended Dose (in trouble): 100–500 mg twice daily, up to 500–1,000 mg twice daily orally but only under the guidance of a health-care professional.

　　50–100 mg IM (intramuscular injection)

Maximum safe level: Unknown. Not necessary to take more than 1–2 grams a day, which is known to be safe.

Contraindications: None for oral doses. Intramuscular injections of thiamine can cause anaphylactic reaction in very rare cases.

Vitamin A

Vitamin A is intimately involved with the creation and maintenance of tissue, especially brain tissue. It is fat soluble, and the brain is composed largely of fat. Warriors who smoke have a special need for vitamin A, as it aids in the repair and replacement of damaged respiratory tissue. In a study of Norwegian fishermen who smoked heavily, 25,000 IU a day of vitamin A in the natural fish liver oil form reduced the lung cancer rate so much that if you didn't know better, you'd think they were non-smokers.

I prefer to use the real, natural vitamin A from fish liver oil. Beta-carotene, a vitamin A precursor found in vegetables and fruits, must be converted in our bodies to become usable vitamin A. This conversion doesn't always happen, especially in people who are sick or older, or who have poor thyroid function, or who live in cold weather. For this reason, I recommend fish liver oil to most of my patients.

When I buy vitamin A capsules, I bite open a capsule to taste the oil. Fresh vitamin A oil is bland and almost tasteless. The older the oil, the fishier it tastes, and the more it has oxidized and become rancid.

Take 25,000 IU of natural vitamin A from fish liver oil five days a week, skipping weekends.

Vitamin A

RDA: 5,000 IU

Recommended Dose (general): 10,000 IU

Recommended Dose (in trouble): 25,000 IU

Maximum safe level: 30,000 IU

Contraindications: Don't take vitamin A supplements during pregnancy.

Pyridoxine (Vitamin B6)

Vitamin B6 is important for metabolizing protein, so Warriors on a high-protein diet must be especially sure to get enough. It is also key in the biochemical transformation of the amino acid tryptophan into the neurotransmitter serotonin. Warriors in trouble are often low in serotonin, so again this is a boost they can use. In a combination of both benefits, the richest sources of tryptophan are the animal proteins, which are meat, fish, chicken, eggs, and milk.

Vitamin B6 is crucial in the brain. The transmission of sensory information to the brain requires B6. Moreover, it increases the intensity and recall of dreams, heightening mental images. Transmission in the brain of light, sound, and heat depends on B6.

The RDA for B6 is 2 mg a day. Preventive and therapeutic doses range from 5 to 1,000 mg daily. If you take more than 50 mg a day—which would only be in trouble—you should do so along with two tablespoons of brewer's yeast, a good B complex, 400 mg of chelated magnesium, 80 mg of zinc sulfate, and 80 mg of riboflavin (another B vitamin).

Vitamin B6

RDA (men): 2 mg
(women): 1–6 mg

Recommended Dose (general): 10 mg

Recommended Dose (in trouble): 100–200 mg (with brewer's yeast, B-complex, magnesium, zinc, and riboflavin, as described in the text)

Contraindications: If you're taking L-dopa (as for Parkinson's), check with a doctor before using vitamin B6 supplements.

Cobalamin (Vitamin B12)

Deficiency of vitamin B12 has been associated with violent behavior, as well as organic brain syndrome, paranoia, and depression. And you don't have to have levels low enough to count as anemia before you experience negative effects. Vitamin B12 is stored in the liver—enough to last three to five years.

Dietary lack of vitamin B12 is rare, but since we get the nutrient almost exclusively from animal products (meat, poultry, fish, eggs, and dairy products), strict vegetarians need to be particularly careful to get enough. Furthermore, many people, particularly as they age, don't have enough stomach intrinsic factor to absorb the B12 they do take in. Brewer's yeast is a good option, as it is rich in vitamin B12. Fortified cereals can also do the trick, and the B12 they contain is much more absorbable for everyone. Or, of course, you can take standard supplements.

Still, most balanced Warriors won't require heavy-duty B12 supplementation. For them, a small oral dose will do. For the type in trouble, however, B12 injections can be invaluable.

Vitamin B12

RDA: 6 mcg daily (taken orally)

Recommended Dose (in balance): 1,000 mcg daily (taken orally or sublingually)

Recommended Dose (in trouble): 1,000 mcg by injection every 3–4 days for 2–3 months

Maximum safe level: Unknown

Contraindications: None

INTERVENTIONS—FOR TIMES OF TROUBLE ONLY

The supplements in this section are for rebalancing when you are in trouble and are not usually used daily over the long term. Once you've gotten your diet under control and given it a little time to work, you probably won't find them necessary. For information on combining natural and prescription treatments, see Chapter 3: The Stoic (p. 102).

INTERVENTION	DAILY DOSE
B12	1,000 mcg (1 ml) injected every 3–4 days
Amino Acids	
Tryptophan	1–9 g (1–3 g for sleep)
Methionine	500 mg–2 g (in trouble)
Herbs	
Green Tea	2–4 cups a day (no more than 300 mg caffeine)

Tryptophan

Low levels of the amino acid tryptophan in the diet have been associated with aggressive behavior in animal studies. Rats are more aggressive toward mice when they are fed a diet almost completely lacking in tryptophan. Another study showed that rats on a low-tryptophan diet (resulting in brain levels 41 percent lower than normal) fought more, were more sensitive to pain, and were more aggressive. A study of monkeys on a diet deficient in tryptophan showed increased aggression. Monkeys who received tryptophan became less aggressive, less vigilant, and less hyperactive. The tryptophan was found to be approximately as effective as prescription antidepressants (SSRIs) and worked best on pathological, rather than normal, aggression. The higher the state of arousal it was applied to, the greater difference the tryptophen made.

As for humans, countries with less tryptophan in their food supply have higher murder rates, even when controlled for social and cultural differences. Countries with diets centered on corn (which is low in tryptophan compared to other grains) also have relatively high rates of homicide.

Tryptophan is a precursor to serotonin. Low serotonin has been associated with violent behavior, which most likely explains tryptophan's effectiveness. When diets low in tryptophan have been used to lower brain tryptophan and serotonin in normal humans, the results have been increased aggression and low mood. (Low serotonin may also predispose people to alcohol abuse and hypoglycemia, which in turn are connected to increased violence, creating yet another vicious circle of negative effects.)

Tryptophan supplements have been proven to reduce abnormally aggressive behavior, especially behavior connected to depression, even in the most extreme cases. Alcoholics with low tryptophan levels showed increasing aggression and depression the lower the levels got. A study of hospitalized aggressive psychiatric patients showed that those given tryptophan had less need for antipsychotics and sedatives. In another study, schizophrenics with a history of aggression who took tryptophan improved compared to those taking a placebo.

Tryptophan

Recommended dose: 1–9 g (1–3 g for sleep)

Maximum safe level: 12 g daily (a level used to treat mania, and not usually necessary for Warriors)

Contraindications: Don't drive immediately after taking tryptophan, at least until you are familiar with how it affects you, as it may make you drowsy. Do not take tryptophan without consulting with your physician if you are taking antidepressant drugs, as they may act synergistically and raise serotonin *too* high.

Methionine

Warriors also benefit from the amino acid methionine, which lowers histamine. It must be taken with pyridoxine (vitamin B6) or else it could make harmful homocysteine.

Methionine

Recommended dose in trouble: 500 mg–2 g a day

Contraindications: High levels (20 g a day) can cause hallucinations in some schizophrenics.

Green Tea

Green tea is the same plant as black tea, except it isn't fermented. While all tea may have health benefits, green tea, in particular, is helpful. It provides a mild stimulant, not as severe as coffee.

A cup of green tea has 80 to 140 mg of polyphenols and 50 mg of caffeine (though you can buy decaf). You can also get capsules of green tea extract. Look for the ones standardized to 60–80 percent polyphenols.

Green Tea

Recommended dose: 2–4 cups a day (no more than 300 mg caffeine)

Maximum safe level: 4–5 cups a day

Contraindications: None. Possible side effects include hyperacidity, gastric irritation, reduced appetite, constipation, and diarrhea. Adding milk can reduce or avoid these side effects, as it binds the chlorogenic acid and other tannins in tea.

Mind/Body and Lifestyle Changes

The key problem for the Warrior in trouble is strengthening control of the outer "civilized" brain over the inner "primitive" brain. You don't want to alter your fundamental Warrior nature, of course, but try on traits from some other types every now and then. You may find some strategies you'll want to make use of, although they may take some practice if they aren't your first instinctive choice. Check the types next to—and directly across from—yours on the pie chart (p. 28).

Plan ahead. The happy Warrior balances the thrill of spontaneity with the Guardian's prudent planning for the future. Try this out by doing something as simple as deciding what you'll do next Saturday, or Sunday, or as forward thinking as opening and funding a retirement account. Give up smoking or break some other bad (but temporarily enjoyable) habit in the interests of your future health. Decide on your summer vacation plans well before the weather warms up. Wear a watch or keep a pocket calendar for a week (if you don't already)—and follow it.

Do unto others. Warriors are very good at taking care of themselves. That can lead to the occasional blind spot when it comes to caring for others. Making a conscious effort to be empathic and/or compassionate helps maintain a healthy balance. Try saying yes the next time someone asks you for a favor. Be on the lookout for a time when someone in your life needs a hand (a household chore, moving, child care, a ride to the airport)—and volunteer to help out. Do an anonymous good deed. Make a donation to charity. Ask someone else what they think before you make a decision that could affect them (whether it is just what to make for dinner, or whether or not to take a new job).

Take your time and do it right. Pick a project, and complete it with a Guardian mantra—"If something is worth doing, it's worth doing well"— running through your head. Follow it as best you can. Dot the I's and cross the T's before turning in your next work assignment. Finish something you started long ago and left half done. Make dinner for your family, and clean up afterward.

Study. Strengthen your cognitive brain by learning something complex or something that requires concentration.

Slow down. I almost always recommend exercise to my patients, but Warriors may actually need rest. (Not that they don't need exercise—they do—but they tend to be so active that they sometimes overdo it.) Slow-moving sports or games requiring patience, discipline, and control also stimulate the cognitive brain. Play chess. Take a yoga class. Try golf. Walk instead of run.

Lengthen your fuse. The next time someone does something that annoys you, try ignoring it or walking away rather than confronting him. When you're bursting to say something, silently count to ten before opening your mouth. Save an angry e-mail until the next day, and see if you still want to send it.

Look inside. Warriors are usually outwardly directed, so incorporating elements from a more inner-directed, quiet lifestyle is another way to achieve some balance. Keep a journal for a month. Listen to a relaxation tape. Try meditation.

GROUP THERAPY

Warriors can benefit greatly from group therapy, because (along with the specific issues addressed, whatever they may be) it promotes relatedness and social adaptation.

I learned a lot about the Warrior type when I was running a prison rehab unit full of them. I conducted a group therapy session for them for several hours every day. These were convicted criminals I was working with—Warriors in trouble—although most were incarcerated for "victimless crimes" (mostly dealing drugs to support their addictions). Although their moral sense did not necessarily line up with the legal system's, there was a rigorous morality nonetheless, and it was accompanied by a clear code of honor. The way the program worked was that the inmates themselves decided who had made enough progress to be "promoted" through the ranks. When they reached the highest rank, they were eligible for parole. Essentially, they voted themselves and each other out of prison. They were ruthlessly honest with each other, and I never had to step in to stop the release of someone clearly not ready for it. It was an extraordinary democracy, but it worked. An astounding 96 percent of our parolees were still clean six months after release from prison—compared to 14 percent in the standard government program at the time.

6

The
Star

The Star type is much less prevalent than the Stoic type, though Stars also experience depression when they are out of balance biochemically. Possibly 2 percent of adult Americans are Stars. Generally cheerful, highly creative, and driven—a "mover and shaker" who gets a lot of joy out of life—a Star in trouble too easily flares up and burns out, in repeated cycles of days, weeks, or months that take a heavy emotional toll. When they are strong enough to interfere with daily functions, these dramatic and cyclical mood swings are identified in textbooks as "bipolar affective disorder" (formerly "manic depression"). But for the Star in balance or merely in minor trouble, the notion of moody or "up and down" might apply. I prefer the imagery of the Star, as it reflects the brightness, heat, and beauty of the profile—in both the celestial and celebrity senses. It also hints at the vast darkness surrounding each point of light—and the white-hot core—making deviations in either direction problematic. But in balance, its beauty is unmatched.

It has taken several years of intense personal scrutiny for me to conclude that I am a Star. That's because I seem to follow extremely long cycles—years long. I never get to the outermost extremes, thanks to keeping my brain supplied with the nutrients it needs and avoiding substances with toxic effects. But I definitely have long swings through "high" periods when I am much more active and productive, alternating with lengthy stretches of time when I am more quiet and introspective.

Within that broad cycle of years, there are, of course, many ups and downs on a more frequent basis, but the overarching pattern is clear. In one earlier active or "up" span, I testified before the United States Senate as an expert in nutrition and mental illness, founded a national medical society, and wrote my first book, all within the space of a few years. A quiet period followed immediately after, during which I just wasn't taking part in the public sphere and spent most of my energy on my family and my own internal and spiritual life.

More recently, I've been back in another active period, having organized two major nutritional health conferences and written another book. But these years followed another quiet period, which I was thrown into after the trauma of my house burning down abruptly ended another active period. These last few years, I've felt drawn to making things happen again, in my life and in the world around me.

I'm more physically active in my "up" periods, with much more energy, and less physical in quiet times. There's a difference in how much time I spend socializing, too, and I withdraw from the world to spend time in introspection, with little interest in a social life, during my quiet periods.

I think all that is quite normal. I cherish the quiet "inner" times as much as the busy "outer" times. I wouldn't want a drug to erase any of it—I don't want to miss a thing. But vitamins are fine, even life-saving, in helping with mood crises. Unlike drugs, nutrients don't interfere with the critical experience. Instead, they simply give your system the biochemical strength to function at your highest level.

Not all Stars make dramatic about-faces in moods seemingly at the drop of a hat. And if you are on an extended cycle, it may be harder to identify yourself as a Star. Of course, we all have aspects of more than one profile in us. But as I've said, one in particular usually predominates. It is all relative. You don't have to be starting companies or appearing on David Letterman to be in an active period. A new job, an addition to the family, or any of the milestones in your life count too. For Stars, these milestones tend to clump together in time, when you take a look at the long view.

You've already met, in the first chapter, one of the Stars I've worked with—Sarah, the painter struggling with depression and infertility. Typical of a Star, she is a charismatic leader and a dominant personality. When she sets her mind to something, she gets it done, and it is often big ideas she sets her mind to. Creativity is also a big part of her life, which is common in Stars.

Though Sarah's "up" periods were always pleasant and never out of control (her problem being the long low points in between them), the danger for many Stars with imbalanced brain chemistry is that their great energy and enthusiasm can veer over into dramatic excess. That's when symptoms like holding themselves in inordinately high esteem, or jumping from one grandiose scheme to the next, show up. They might also be excessively talkative, distractible, and uninhibited, and complain angrily of the ineptitude all around them. Others frequently notice their lack of concentration, racing speech, and poor judgment. Troubled Stars may suddenly need very little sleep because they are so full of their joyous misguided manic excitement. They may also increase their involvement in work or social activities, or plunge into spending sprees, sexual indiscretions, or misguided financial decisions. They feel euphoric, elated, and invincible—good things in moderation, but for the Star in trouble these emotions pass the point of all reason. Stars out of balance don't recognize the downsides, however, and believe they are functioning at their peak. The phrase "delusions of grandeur" must have been coined with a Star in mind.

Perhaps because her case was relatively mild, Sarah's depression looked much like a Stoic's. Most Stars, by contrast, tend toward big, dramatic, splashy depression (not the "smiling depression" so many Stoics manifest) when their chemistry tips out of balance. Stars in trouble may sleep too much (or too little), withdraw from society, lose interest in the things that normally engage them, feel pessimistic, and act irritable, just as Stoics in trouble do. The hopelessness, low self-esteem, lack of motivation, and avoidance of relationships will look much the same. But unlike Stoics, Stars will

Star Profile: Winston Churchill

No one could set out to save the world from 1,000 years of tyranny without at least something of the Star in themselves. Winston Churchill was a Star through and through—big visions, big personality, big career. Stars are often leaders, though no doubt it took an especially intense one to lead the entire free world—into combat, no less. Churchill loved the grand things in life—fine cigars and excellent alcohol among them—and often indulged to (what for most people would be) excess. Still, he was extremely functional when he was "up," and though he was famous for his short fuse, he did not seem to ever get out of control.

On the other hand, at times he took to bed for a week or more, fed by a nurse as if he were an invalid, cursing his "Black Dog"—depression. Listen to his existential gloom even on an occasion when he led his country to a negotiation table: "We are only specs of dust, that have settled in the night on a map of the world." These bouts of deep depression plagued him all his life. As a young man he described the darkness: "When I was young, for two or three years the light faded out of the picture. I did my work. I sat in the House . . . but black depression settled on me. . . . I don't like standing near the edge of a platform when an express train is passing. I like to stand right back and if possible to get a pillar between me and the train. I don't like to stand beside the side of a ship and look down into the water. A second's action would end everything. A few drops of desperation. And yet I don't want to go out of the world at all in such moments."

One historian concluded that Churchill retreated from adversity into depression at times, and at other times even his simplest actions were carried out in "typically grand" ways. These dramatic contrasts are hallmarks of the Star. Consider the string of descrip-

(continued)

Star Profile: Winston Churchill *(continued)*

tions employed by another historian: energetic, impetuous, extravagant, sybaritic, difficult, obsessive, temperamental, petulant, blustery, sensitive, and insecure. And that's just one paragraph's worth! Whether dark or light, Churchill's moods, like a Star's, tended to be, as this historian put it, "overblown."

be sure to tell everyone around them all about their misery. Stars are also vulnerable to attacks of rage, fierce defensiveness, feelings of persecution, and hostility—sometimes even hallucinations—usually with no "reason" (other than unbalanced brain chemistry). Failing to finish projects that were started with much fanfare is a specialty of a Star careening from high to low.

Psychiatry would label the Star in trouble with "bipolar depression" or "manic depression." But of course, most Stars are *not* in trouble most of the time, or at least not drastically so. Most Stars would tend to think of themselves as "moody," perhaps, and recognize rather up-and-down behavior.

Psychiatry understands unipolar depression reasonably thoroughly, but understands bipolar disorders less fully. That's because traditional psychiatry is overly pessimistic about these two states, viewing them as entirely negative, without recognizing their positive aspects. So there has been less success treating the bipolar depression of Stars than the unipolar type of Stoics in trouble. That may be because the moods are so different, and the chemistry underlying them is so distinct (as we'll see in the next section), making the necessary pharmacological response more complicated.

It may also be because the mania feels so good. What Star would want to give up the rush of an "up" phase? The fortunate ones, like Sarah, enjoy the high without getting out of control. Her problem, then, when she was in trouble, was simpler by half: She had only to correct the imbalances resulting in depression to return to her best self.

The good news is that the possibility is there for *any* Star to reclaim all the heady exuberance of his profile *with no fear* of swinging either into de-

Type	General Traits	Beneficial Aspects	Harmful Aspects	Vulnerabilities
Stars	Energetic (and energizing)	Are movers and shakers.	Are melodramatic.	Stars in trouble tend to get
	Loving	Persevere.	Dominate others.	depressed and/
	Intense	See the big picture.	Abuse others.	or manic (as a
	Passionate	Are natural leaders.	Exhaust others.	defense against
	Intuitive	Have big ideas.	Are self-centered.	depression).
	Creative	Have high self-esteem.	Are impulsive.	Star's
	Exuberant	Can count Winston	Get grandiose.	depression is
	Charismatic	Churchill as one of	Are excessively	always drama-
	Dominant	their own.	talkative.	tic (unlike the
	Dramatic		Are easily distractible.	Stoic's).
			Lose all inhibition.	
			Act superior.	
			Show poor judgment.	
			Are hostile.	
			Lack follow-through.	

pression or the excesses of unbridled impulse. With balanced brain chemistry, the Star is perhaps the perfect example of what can happen when the inner ("old") and outer ("new") brain work perfectly in concert. With excellent neurotransmitter communication supported by good nutrition, the two areas can do their work completely and thoroughly, and Stars can feel fulfilled that the deepest inner desires of their souls are in harmony with their outer cortical functions of thought and conscience. Human brains are unique in this two-part design, and using the capabilities it gives us to the greatest extent possible is to be most fully human.

Dietary Guidelines

The proper diet will help you be the best Star you can be, maximizing all the positive traits and minimizing any negative tendencies. Supplements and mind/body techniques will help, too, but must be built upon the solid foundation of a diet that is healthy for your type. Once your body is in balance, you won't need to be as strict with your diet. On the other hand, when you are out of balance, a more rigid approach will help you stabilize. Stars must pay attention to which way they fall out of balance in order to know how to bring themselves back into balance.

The basic high-protein, limited-carbohydrate hypoglycemic diet laid out in Chapter 3 (The Stoic) would serve adequately for Stars—or anyone with hypoglycemia. Even more important than the balance of macronutrients and the specific foods you eat is the *wholeness* of what you eat.

The body burns carbohydrates quickly—in about an hour to an hour and a half—while fats and proteins take around five hours. For Stars in trouble, the slower burn of proteins and fats can slow down someone in a manic state and help keep his moods on an even keel.

I also recommend that Stars add serotonin-promoting foods during down times—and avoid them in manic phases, when serotonin levels are already too high. Even more important is eliminating stimulants (caffeine and sugar prime among them) during mania, as they can cause or worsen the manic flight of ideas and other negative symptoms. (Drugs like cocaine and amphetamines, which are also stimulants, can be even more damaging to a Star than to other types for this reason.) Additionally, a Star in trouble must avoid alcohol. For one thing, it is a depressant. For another, its effect

Essential Foods	Danger Foods
Serotonin-promoting foods when you feel down.	Serotonin-promoting foods, caffeine, and other stimulants (like sugar) when manic.
Fats and proteins to calm a manic mood.	Alcohol.
Fruits and other natural sugars to lift a blue mood.	Common allergens: Wheat, corn, coffee, milk, eggs, potatoes, oranges, beef, pork, yeast, tomatoes, peanuts, and soy. (Food allergies are common in Stars; you may want to be tested to find out what you in fact react to.)

Case in Point

One of my patients often arrived for his sessions singing at the top of his lungs (loud enough that I was worried about disturbing my neighbors). He was coming for help with his anger and extreme antisocial behavior (he once approached a stranger on the street and shoved her, for example). He was a talented and promising college student, but now was on the verge of flunking out if he didn't do something to earn expulsion first. Whenever I saw him, he was always toting a large cup of coffee or a liter bottle of cola.

I recommended vitamin E to calm and relax him and, because he was deficient in folic acid, a B-complex supplement along with extra folic acid. I counseled him on cleaning up his diet, but my main concern was that he cut out caffeine in order to gain control of his behavior again.

As soon as he cut back, it was clear he was one of those people who are particularly sensitive to caffeine. His improvement was rapid and dramatic. He was no longer irrational or unpredictably angry. As he experienced the connection between his out-of-control behavior and his caffeine intake, he cut back on it even more. Recognizing how he let coffee take him out of control allowed him to learn to limit it.

He went on to become a straight-A student at a prestigious graduate school and even learned how to manage some caffeine (he did really love coffee)—drinking it occasionally with meals, and only when he was otherwise stable. His diet improved, too, with fewer "whites," but it remained far from perfect. For him, it was all about the caffeine.

on blood sugar is the same as having pure sugar. It is metabolized very rapidly as a carbohydrate. Alcohol also interferes with nutrient absorption from food, especially thiamine (vitamin B1) and cobalamin (vitamin B12), and, to top it all off, causes dehydration (by promoting the diuretic effect well known to anyone who has ever had too much to drink), which can result in the lowering of levels of crucial minerals.

The Star Diet

This eating program is designed to balance the Star's brain chemistry. It isn't meant as a weight-loss diet, though in combination with regular exercise, it should help you get to and stay at a healthy weight, as well as stay healthy in general. You don't have to keep track of calories or fat grams or numbers of carbohydrates or anything else except the number of servings you have each day from a few key categories. And here they are:

- 5–7 small meals a day
- 4–5 servings of protein
- 2 servings of legumes
- 1 serving nuts and seeds (optional)
- 5–8 servings of vegetables
- 2–3 servings of fruit
- 4–5 servings whole grains

This holds as a maintenance diet for when you are in balance, or for rebalancing yourself if you've fallen toward depression. If you veer toward manic instead, there are a few caveats:

- Trade in some or all of the fruits for vegetables, and make sure you're getting healthy fats along with your protein.
- Eliminate serotonin-promoting foods during these times (avocado, banana, eggplant, pineapple, plum, tomato, walnut).
- Avoid stimulants like caffeine and sugar.
- Cut out alcohol.

The chart that follows summarizes the best food choices for Stars in balance. A chart somewhat altered for Stars tipping toward depression and another customized for Stars tipping toward mania follow.

FOR STARS IN BALANCE

FOOD	BEST CHOICES	GOOD CHOICES	AVOID
Animal Protein (4–5 servings)	milk and dairy products beef sardines chicken (enriched with DHA) lamb eggs turkey	poultry fish caviar pork salmon tuna herring halibut	processed dairy and meats
Vegetables (5–8 servings)	seaweed (hijiki, nori, and kombu) peas alfalfa sprouts carrots spinach asparagus lettuce onions garlic red pepper	Brussels sprouts collards green peppers kale mustard greens parsley mushrooms broccoli cabbage cauliflower potatoes tomatoes	canned or frozen vegetables, esp. if they contain sugar, EDTA, or preservatives
Fruit (2–3 servings)	lemons oranges cantaloupe	apricots berries melon cherries limes guava grapefruit kiwi mangoes papaya strawberries	canned or frozen fruit
Whole Grains (4–5 servings)	whole grain bread whole grain cereals brown rice shredded wheat cereal oatmeal	wheat corn	white flour white rice

FOOD	BEST CHOICES	GOOD CHOICES	AVOID
Legumes (2 servings)	soy black beans pinto beans garbanzo beans (chickpeas) lentils navy beans lima beans kidney beans	tofu	
Nuts and Seeds (1 serving, optional)	almonds walnuts pecans Brazil nuts	pistachios cashews sunflower seeds pumpkin seeds (and other squash seeds) sesame seeds	Peanuts
Sweeteners	maple syrup honey		white sugar
Beverages	mineral water green tea ginseng tea		caffeinated drinks (including coffee, tea, sodas, and sodas)
Condiments and Seasonings	lecithin		yeast

FOR STARS TIPPING TOWARD DEPRESSION

FOOD	BEST CHOICES	GOOD CHOICES	AVOID
Animal Protein (4–5 servings)	milk and dairy products eggs beef sardines chicken (enriched with DHA) salmon tuna turkey herring halibut	poultry lamb fish pork caviar	

FOOD	BEST CHOICES	GOOD CHOICES	AVOID
Vegetables (5–8 servings)	avocados eggplant seaweed (hijiki, nori, and kombu) peas alfalfa sprouts carrots spinach asparagus lettuce onion red pepper	Brussels sprouts collards garlic kale mustard greens parsley peppers mushrooms broccoli cabbage cauliflower potatoes tomatoes	canned or frozen vegetables
Fruit (2–3 servings)	pineapple plums bananas lemons cantaloupe oranges	apricots berries melons cherries limes guava grapefruit kiwi mangoes papaya strawberries	canned or frozen fruit, esp. in sugar syrup
Whole Grains (4–5 servings)	whole grain bread whole grain cereals brown rice shredded wheat cereal oatmeal	whole wheat corn	white flour white rice
Legumes (2 servings)	tofu black beans pinto beans garbanzo beans (chickpeas) lentils navy beans lima beans kidney beans		sugar-laced canned beans
Nuts and Seeds (1 serving, optional)	almonds walnuts	pistachios cashews sunflower seeds	peanuts

FOOD	BEST CHOICES	GOOD CHOICES	AVOID
		pumpkin seeds (and other squash seeds) sesame seeds pecans Brazil nuts	
Sweeteners	maple syrup honey		white sugar
Beverages	mineral water green tea ginseng tea		caffeinated drinks (including coffee, tea, sodas, and diet sodas)
Condiments and Seasonings	lecithin		yeast

FOR STARS TIPPING TOWARD MANIA

FOOD	BEST CHOICES	GOOD CHOICES	AVOID
Animal Protein (4–5 servings)	sardines canned sardines (with bones) chicken (enriched with DHA) salmon canned salmon (with bones) turkey herring halibut	poultry lamb fish caviar codfish pork tuna	milk and dairy products eggs beef
Vegetables (6-11 servings)	seaweed (hijiki, nori, and kombu) alfalfa sprouts broccoli cabbage carrots spinach asparagus lettuce onions cauliflower peas	beets beet greens Brussels sprouts collards garlic kale mustard greens parsley peppers radishes mushrooms turnip greens dark green leafy vegetables	potatoes tomatoes avocados eggplant tomatoes

FOOD	BEST CHOICES	GOOD CHOICES	AVOID
Fruit (1 serving, optional)	lemons cantaloupe oranges	apricots berries melon cherries limes guava grapefruit kiwi mangoes papaya strawberries	bananas pineapple .red plums
Whole Grains (4–5 servings)	whole grain bread whole grain cereal brown rice shredded wheat cereal oatmeal		wheat corn
Legumes (2 servings)		black beans pinto beans garbanzo beans (chickpeas) lentils navy beans lima beans kidney beans	soy
Nuts and Seeds (1 serving, optional)	almonds	pistachios cashews sunflower seeds pumpkin seeds (and other squash seeds) pecans Brazil nuts sesame seeds	peanuts walnuts
Sweeteners	maple syrup		refined sugars
Beverages	mineral water green tea (decaffeinated) ginseng tea chamomile tea		alcohol caffeinated drinks (including coffee, tea, sodas, and diet sodas)
Condiments and Seasonings	lecithin		yeast

Brain Chemistry Markers

SEROTONIN

For a Star in trouble, just as for the Stoic, serotonin and cortisol are the markers to watch out for. In depression, serotonin is low and cortisol is high, while in mania, the reverse is true: serotonin is high and cortisol is low. If you are a Star who feels you may be in trouble, talk to your doctor about having your levels tested. (See Chapter 4: The Guardian for a full rundown of the components of a thorough workup.)

As we saw in the last chapter, adequate brain serotonin (normal being between 5 and 20 mgc/dcl) means good cheer, while low levels spark depression. Stars have an additional danger when they are in trouble: Serotonin can rise too high (over 20 mgc/dl), causing manic symptoms.

CORTISOL

Cortisol, the main adrenal hormone and a general stress indicator, follows the opposite pattern. It is high (30 mgc/dl or more) in severe depression, since a depressed mental state *is* a serious stressor. On the other hand, when Stars are in trouble in a manic phase, cortisol is low (less than 3–6 mcg/dl) because they feel *good*, and despite any actual problems, they aren't stressed about them. They wade so deep in denial, they aren't even aware of them. For me, this phenomenon of how thoroughly mania defends against depression—to the point where it even alters biochemistry—is a reminder of how powerfully important the mind is in effecting change in the body.

I seldom have my patients get their cortisol levels tested. Since it is just a reflection of a state of stress, it is usually clear from how they appear—and how they say they feel—whether or not they are stressed, so I don't want them to have to spend their money on an official test. But it is an option, and sometimes it can clarify a situation.

I use the test for serotonin more routinely, as a biochemical marker for mood states—low in depression, high in mania. Although it can be expensive, most insurance plans should cover it. Since we are working with nutrients with few if any significant side effects, simply trying the different treatments is an option if the cost of testing is prohibitive.

The Cortisol Roller Coaster

I was still a medical student working a summer job with the famous New York Hospital endocrinologist Peter Stokes, M.D., when a patient taught me about how cortisol levels shift in manic depression. When I met him, Montgomery had very, very high cortisol levels—higher than those I'd seen with adrenal gland tumors. He was severely depressed, sitting in posh Payne Whitney Psychiatric Clinic, a retreat for New York's super-rich, upset and crying over the mess he claimed to have made of his life.

Just days later, Montgomery was happy and bubbling, chuckling over a great deal he'd made over the weekend: He'd bought not one, not two, but *three* new Thunderbird convertibles. Clearly he'd flipped from depression into mania. When I checked his cortisol level, it had plummeted. His body wasn't experiencing much stress, so it didn't need to produce a lot of cortisol.

It was a powerful biochemical lesson for me. Other people might have felt some stress signing the papers for just one new car without careful research and comparison shopping. Not Monty.

It was also a lesson to me about labeling certain behavior through my own biased perspective. Thinking that buying three cars in one go was inappropriate (to say the least), I'm sure I noted something in his record about impaired judgment—just the kind of thing we were being taught to be on the lookout for in manic-depressive patients. I was unable to think outside the box the way he was, so I missed the main point. Looking back, I can understand Monty better as a Star (not just labeled as a manic-depressive), and I've wondered: If he did indeed keep those cars stored in garages and drove them minimally, as he explained his plan to me, those 1962 beauties would be priceless classics now. Was his judgment really impaired just because no one else could see, as he im-

(continued)

> **The Cortisol Roller Coaster** *(continued)*
>
> mediately did, that those cars were going to be classics? He did,
> after all, have the money to spend. Maybe he had a real vision.
> Maybe he was just ahead of his time. Maybe he'd actually made a
> really smart deal.

ZINC, COPPER, AND MAGNESIUM

The other brain chemistry markers for a Stoic in trouble (histamine, copper, zinc, and magnesium) are also relevant for a Star in trouble in the "down" part of the cycle, and may be worth testing for. High copper is especially common. (See Chapter 3: The Stoic.) There is no evidence, however, that copper levels change with moods the way the neurotransmitters do, and there is no evidence linking low copper levels with mania.

HISTAMINE

Histamine is often low in mania (as it is often high in depression). Low histamine manics are grandiose, overly optimistic, and easily deluded because they are so caught up in their own thoughts that their judgment is often faulty. This test can be difficult to come by.

> **Case in Point**
>
> Tony's serotonin was completely normal, but his histamine was
> too low. Normal is often between 4 and 7 mcg/dl, and his was just
> 3.2. The severe mood swings he experienced were classically those
> of someone with low histamine. He described getting overexcited
> and lapsing easily into fantasy life. He spoke too hurriedly, flitted
> from one idea to the next, and even lost a degree of physical coor-
>
> *(continued)*

Case in Point *(continued)*

dination. He slept little. He would stay up all night studying complicated scientific texts, and forget to shower or shave, oblivious (or indifferent) to the effect it was having on his work.

When I first saw Tony he was depressed, lacking in confidence, and a bit befuddled. (That's the way it always is with Stars, who rarely seek help when they are manic and overly optimistic.) He kept meticulous records of his interactions with the medical establishment, and he worked at the various therapies recommended to him over the years earnestly and with dedication—like the Eagle Scout and straight-A student he had been. When I think back to the "old" Tony, I'm still reminded of the Saturday Night Live character Stuart Smalley, with the corny motto, "I'm good enough, I'm smart enough, and—gosh darn it—people like me!"

Tony's serotonin level was completely normal, though I'd been expecting it to be low, reflecting his current depression, or even high, a reminder or predictor of the last or next manic phase. The vitamin panel I ordered was unremarkable—everything came back "normal." He was generally low in minerals and had a markedly disturbed copper/zinc ratio, with a toxically high copper level.

He'd already been diagnosed with hypoglycemia, though no particular treatment had ever been recommended. In reviewing the results from the hypoglycemia test, I saw the typical Star pattern—very high elevation followed by a rapid and deep decline below baseline. As with so many Stars, Tony's blood sugar was as volatile as his emotional state.

I started by explaining the basic hypoglycemic diet. I also gave Tony a regimen to raise his histamine levels: cobalamin (vitamin B12) (via injection, to ensure absorption) and folic acid supplements. He took zinc to balance his copper levels and a B-complex

(continued)

Case in Point *(continued)*

supplement to support his adrenal gland and fight fatigue. He took additional pantothenic acid (vitamin B5), pyridoxine (vitamin B6), niacin (vitamin B3), and vitamin C.

Tony had been on very high doses of lithium for years, as well as tranquilizers. I helped him taper down his doses slowly, over many months. After about a year, with a properly nourished brain, he was taking only an eighth of the tranquilizers he'd been using before, and a third of the lithium—with no loss in its effectiveness.

During his years on the drugs, Tony developed a weight problem. That's a common side effect of lithium, which depresses the thyroid, which controls metabolism. On top of that, the tranquilizers increased his appetite and made him crave junk foods. So not only was he overeating, he was gorging on unhealthy foods that kept his brain chemistry out of balance and deepened his dependence on the drugs. But as he started to get well, he began to lose weight. Eating less junk food eventually cut his cravings for it. Better eating habits allowed him to reduce his drug dosage. Lower doses of drugs lessened the negative side effects. Tony was on a cycle again—but this time a positive one, with each beneficial change reinforcing the other.

Within two months of starting treatment, Tony's zinc and copper were in balance, relieving his depression and calming his agitation. Within five months, his blood sugar was normalized. After a year, a repeat vitamin panel showed high levels of vitamins (where they had been just "normal" before). He was feeling so good, I took this as another argument to take "normal" results with a grain of salt. For Tony, "normal" wasn't enough. To experience the best of health, his body required "high" levels. A year and a half into his treatment, his serotonin remained normal, a reminder that

(continued)

Case in Point *(continued)*

not every individual shows all the blood chemistry markers typical of his or her condition.

All together, I worked with Tony about three years, until we reached the happy outcome: I never saw him again. And he never called for refills on his prescriptions.

Normal Levels for Brain Chemistry Markers

Serotonin	55–260 ng/ml (nanograms per milliliter)
Histamine	9–141 ng/ml
Cortisol	varies during the day:
	8–26 mg/100 ml in the morning;
	2–18 mg/100 ml in the afternoon;
	<6 mg/100 ml at midnight
Copper	65–155 mcg/dl (normal range varies from lab to lab)
Zinc	60–130 mcg/dl (micrograms per deciliter)
Magnesium	1.3–2.5 meq/L (milliequivalent per liter)

Hypoglycemia

As with nearly all the types, hypoglycemia is the dietary Achilles' heel for Stars in trouble. The average American diet, which is full of sugars and fats and devoid of whole, wholesome food, has left a majority of us malnourished. Hypoglycemia is one of the common signs of malnourishment, and it shows up in every type in trouble. The only difference is in the behavior that results when hypoglycemia throws off the brain chemistry. When that happens, each type runs into trouble in its own characteristic way. For Stars, that means alternating bouts of depression and unchecked elation.

Chapter 3: The Stoic explained the "flat curve" hypoglycemia so many of that type develop. The blood sugar pattern of Stars in trouble is quite different—and also quite fitting. Hypoglycemic Stars usually have what's known as "reactive" hypoglycemia—the most common type in general. That means their blood sugar spikes in reaction to eating sugar—as is normal—then drops far below normal before curving up to normal again. In Stars, however, you'll see a hugely steep increase and a correspondingly harrowing drop, oscillations far more dramatic than in your garden-variety reactive hypoglycemia.

The case that first taught me about the distinctive pattern of hypoglycemia in Stars was a young man named Fred. When he came to see me, he was in the depressed part of his cycle but complained about his "up" moods as well, saying he grew overenamoured with his own apparent cleverness. His judgment would be overtaken by his disproportionately optimistic view of himself. That is just the thing so many Stars find ruinous, as they end up doing things they would never do in a sober state of mind. He was also anxious and tired (though when he wasn't manic he slept reasonably well).

Fred was exceedingly intelligent and an original thinker. I imagine he was well suited to the philosophy Ph.D. program he eventually entered. He was not a big, dynamic, knock-your-socks-off Star. He was relatively mild-mannered (for a Star), but usually charismatic and gregarious. He had all the charm and persuasiveness of the Star, as well as the ability to draw others in with his contagious optimism.

Fred's long-time relationship with a woman had recently disintegrated, and her rejection had wounded him deeply. He felt his job at a photography studio was stressing him out, and he worried about the exposure he was getting there to a variety of chemicals. But he was a good employee (at least when he wasn't over the edge), and he was energetic and organized.

Fred had already been diagnosed as manic-depressive, and in fact had been hospitalized several times. (The one time I saw him in the hospital, where he'd checked in just for testing, he was in the center of a cluster of other patients, strumming his guitar and singing. If I had had any doubts he was a Star, this would have been a confirmation!) His other doctors had prescribed lithium to control his mood swings, but Fred wasn't entirely satisfied with the results. He still felt he didn't have complete clarity in his thinking and that he was too emotional. He also worried about how rough lithium is on the thyroid and kidneys.

A five-hour glucose tolerance test revealed severe reactive hypoglycemia with one of the most extreme blood sugar swings I've ever seen. During the test, his blood sugar rose very high very quickly, but that's normal. It then plunged way below baseline, which is not normal at all. I now know that the wide oscillation in blood sugar—matching the oscillation in mood—is typical of Stars in trouble.

The only other thing of interest revealed by a battery of tests was a generally low level of minerals. He had a shortage of magnesium, a calming mineral, and his copper/zinc ratio was skewed by a high copper level. Copper is a stimulant, and zinc is calming, so along with the other problems an imbalanced ratio can cause (including depression), the mismatch was probably contributing to Fred's overexcited manic states. The rest of his biochemistry was essentially normal. (At the time, the serotonin test was not yet much in use, and I only tested him for it years later. The results were normal—and so was he by then.)

The most important thing for Fred to do was to get his blood sugar under control. His diet was already pretty good. He was a vegetarian who did his grocery shopping exclusively at his local "health" food store. He didn't drink alcohol, though he did drink coffee and tea, and he smoked cigarettes (all stimulants, and all capable of setting off a manic episode). And he did consume plenty of sugar.

Fred quickly adapted to small, frequent meals consisting of more protein and only complex carbohydrates. Getting the protein he needed required a bit more thought since he didn't eat meat, though eggs, dairy, soy products, beans, and other vegetable proteins easily met his needs. He ate three regular meals each day, with two snacks during the day and one at bedtime. He cut back on smoking and caffeine, too, though it took a long time for him to eliminate them altogether.

Fred also committed to getting an hour of exercise a day—he chose walking—for the beneficial effects it has on stabilizing blood sugar. Exercise moves sugar from the bloodstream into cells needing energy, *without* insulin. Since insulin is otherwise required to do that job, exercise effectively gives the pancreas a break, thereby helping stabilize blood sugar levels.

I recommended a basic program of supplements of vitamins A, C, D, E, and the B-complex vitamins. Among its many functions for general health, vitamin C acidifies the blood, making lithium more effective and enabling a lower dose to work. Vitamin C also protects the thyroid gland from the potentially toxic effects of lithium.

Fred also began to take a multimineral supplement in addition to a zinc supplement. I wanted him to get his copper/zinc ratio in balance, of course, but prescribed enough additional zinc to make use of its sedative properties as well. When he eventually went back to school, he quit the job that included chemical exposure (and too much general stress). Repeat testing showed that these steps restored healthy mineral levels in his body.

With all these changes, Fred continued on lithium, though I helped him decrease from the standard dose to a lower dose, about one-quarter of the amount he'd needed before he properly nourished himself and his brain. His mood stayed stable, and he certainly never required another hospitalization. He would come back to see me only once or twice a year, mostly to report how well things were going.

Insomnia

When he was in a manic state, Fred suffered from insomnia—a classic problem for Stars in trouble—and slept only a few hours a night. For those times, I recommended several supplements at bedtime: 400 mg chelated magnesium for its soothing, calming properties; 1,500 mg inositol (a B vitamin usually found in B-complex supplements) to relax him and make him mildly drowsy; and one of his three 200 mg doses for the day of natural vitamin E, also for its subtle muscle-relaxing effect. He drank chamomile and passionflower tea and took 300 mg tryptophan and 500 mg vitamin C. He responded beautifully to these remedies, but in patients who don't respond as well, I also use L-tryptophan (300–3,000 mg).

Then, after several years, as he fully committed to strictly following his new way of eating, and finally kicked his cigarette and caffeine habits, he gave up lithium completely. With his brain chemistry properly balanced, he functioned perfectly well without the medication. He eventually fell in love again, created a successful relationship, and got married. After completing his course of study, he became a minister.

Natural Medicine Solutions

Everything that works for a Stoic in trouble (see Chapter 3) will also work for a troubled Star in the depressed phase, and Stars can refer to that chap-

NATURAL MEDICINE SOLUTIONS FOR DEPRESSION

VITAMINS	MINERALS	AMINO ACIDS	HERBS	FATTY ACIDS
Thiamine (vitamin B1)	Magnesium	Tryptophan	St. John's Wort	DHA
Niacin (vitamin B3)	Cesium	Phenylalanine	Ginseng	
Pantothenic acid (vitamin B5)	Zinc	Tyrosine	Green tea	**ACCESSORY NUTRIENTS**
Folic Acid	Selenium			SAMe
Cobalamin (vitamin B12)	Lithium			
Pyridoxine (vitamin B6)				

NATURAL MEDICINE SOLUTIONS FOR MANIA

VITAMINS	MINERALS	AMINO ACIDS	HERBS	FATTY ACIDS
B-complex	Zinc	Tryptophan	Ginseng	EFAs
Folic Acid	Calcium	5-HTP	Kava	
Vitamin C	Magnesium	Taurine	Chamomile	
	Lithium	Glutamine	Passionflower	
Niacin			Rauwolfia	
Inositol			Serpentina	

ter for details on specific nutrients. Many of the same things work for troubled Stars who are manic—in addition to the supplements only appropriate during the manic phase. The charts on p. 204 summarize all the choices for each phase. Next, we'll go into the daily supplements that are good for Stars, and finally the interventions for Stars in trouble.

DAILY SUPPLEMENTS

The supplement program described here is designed to bring out the best in a Star. It will boost the results of a healthy diet in balancing your brain chemistry, just as a healthy diet will boost the effects of the supplements. The two together are going to work better than either on its own. Where you see a range of doses listed, the lower end is meant for prevention or maintenance, while the higher levels are for when you are in trouble and need something therapeutic. As always, take only what you need.

Daily Supplements

Magnesium: 400 mg daily
Zinc: 30 mg daily
Folic acid: 400 mcg daily
Niacin (vitamin B3): 100 mg daily
Cobalamin (Vitamin B12): 100 mcg daily
Thiamine (vitamin B1): 100 mg daily
Pantothenic acid (Vitamin B5): 100 mg daily
Pyridoxine (Vitamin B6): 10–25 mg daily
Inositol: 500 mg daily
Vitamin C: 500 mg daily

If in trouble (depression), add:
DHA: 4–5 capsules daily
Selenium: 50–300 mcg daily

If in trouble (mania), add:
Calcium: 1 g (1,000 mg) daily
Taurine: 1 g (1,000 mg) daily

> ## Vitamin C
>
> **RDA:** 20 mg
>
> **Recommended dose (in balance):** 500 mg daily
>
> **Recommended dose (in trouble):** 1–50 g daily (see above for specifics)
>
> **Maximum safe level:** Stay 1–2 grams below the level that causes you diarrhea.
>
> **Contraindications:** None

Vitamin C

Stars in trouble exhibit "sub-clinical" scurvy—a mild deficiency in vitamin C. Studies of hospitalized psychiatric patients have shown their vitamin C levels to be low and their absorption of vitamin C to be impaired, even when no other signs of scurvy were present. Another study showed improvements in both manic and depressed patients taking vitamin C (compared to placebo). Yet another study pinpointed the improvements as beginning within three to six hours of taking vitamin C, for both manic and depressed patients.

The body uses vitamin C to regulate nerve impulses and to make the neurotransmitters noradrenaline, adrenaline, dopamine, acetylcholine, and serotonin, which are needed to handle worry, excitement, fear, anger, and other symptoms that can appear in mania or depression. Therefore, a lack of vitamin C can contribute to depression.

Anxiety and excitement increase the rate at which vitamin C is broken down in the body, meaning the body's demand for it may rise when a Star is in trouble, particularly in the manic phase.

In balance, 500 mg a day will help keep you that way. For mild symptoms such as fatigue, pessimism, and worry, take 3 g daily. For moderate symptoms like anxiety, depression, confusion, and insomnia, take 3–10 g daily. (For nighttime sedation, take 1–5 g at bedtime.) For severe symptoms such as mania, severe depression, or a "nervous breakdown," take 3–50 g daily. For drug addiction withdrawal, take 1–2 g every hour. As always for very high doses, you should be under a doctor's care, and using the buffered forms.

B-Complex Vitamins

A balanced B-complex vitamin is de rigueur for any Star, along with 50 or 100 mg of each of the individual B vitamins (see Chapter 3: The Stoic). The B vitamins are essential for normal brain function and a healthy nervous system, and getting all the B vitamins in sufficient quantity is important for stable moods. For Stars, the B vitamins have a lithiumlike effect without any of the harsh side effects.

Folic acid is particularly important for patients who are also taking lithium.

Lack of cobalamin (vitamin B12) can cause mania (or depression or other mental symptoms) three to five years before it causes signs of anemia in the blood, so it is important to get enough of this as well.

Niacin (vitamin B3) is good for fighting depression but is also calming during mania because it supports GABA. A deficiency in niacin can cause mania (or depression), and correcting the deficiency can eliminate the problem.

EFAs (Essential Fatty Acids)

Essential fatty acids (EFAs) are crucial for building the physical brain and for monitoring daily functioning. Furthermore, they are as helpful in mania as they are in depression. Omega-6 may prevent side effects of lithium, especially when taken in combination with potassium. Eggs are an excellent source of EFAs, and just two eggs a day will really build up the adrenals. Soya lecithin supplements are another good source of EFAs.

EFAs are long carbon chain polyunsaturated fats, consisting of linoleic, linolenic, and alpha-linolenic acid. Linoleic acid is the only truly essential EFA. If it is present in the diet, our bodies can use it to manufacture the other necessary fatty acids.

Alpha-linolenic acid is the name of omega-3 fats from land-based, non-marine sources. Most omega-3 fats come from fish oils or are synthesized commercially from algae and plankton. The omega-3 family includes eicosapentaenoic (EPA), docosapentaenoic (DPA), and docosahexaenoic (DHA) acids. The omega-9 fatty acids (arachidonic) are from meats, seaweed, and some dairy products.

EFAs

Recommended dose (in balance): 3–4 capsules daily

Recommended dose (in trouble): 4–6 capsules daily

Maximum safe level: Unknown

Contraindications: Unknown

DHA

In addition to EFAs in general, Stars can benefit from the essential fatty acid DHA (docosahexaenoic acid—not to be confused with the hormone DHEA) is an omega-3 oil found in fish and seaweed. It is particularly helpful to Stars in trouble who are depressed. (For more information, see p. 83 in Chapter 3: The Stoic.)

The eyes and brain use a lot of omega-3 fats, especially DHA. Sixty per-

---

DHA

Recommended dose (in balance): 0–1,000 mg daily

Recommended dose (in trouble): 800–1,250 mg daily

Maximum safe level: Unknown. However, 5,000 mg daily for several months could be harmful.

Contraindications: Diabetics, especially older people, must consult with their doctors before using it, as should infants and pregnant women.

---

cent of the brain is fat, and DHA is the most abundant polyunsaturated fatty acid in both the brain and the retina. Low DHA levels have been linked to several brain chemistry disorders, including depression, and in all these conditions, DHA supplements have had beneficial effects.

Magnesium

Magnesium is a sedative and antidepressant. I tell my patients to use chelated magnesium because it is absorbed more easily by the body.

Magnesium

RDA: 300–600 mg daily

Recommended dose (in balance): 400 mg daily

Recommended dose (in trouble): 600 mg daily

Maximum safe level: Unknown; no need to use more than 600 mg a day, which is known to be safe

Contraindications: Unknown

Selenium

Add selenium to your daily routine if you are sliding toward depression.

Selenium

RDA: 50–200 mcg daily

Recommended dose (in balance): 50–200 mcg daily

Recommended dose (in trouble): 50–300 mcg daily

Maximum safe level: Unknown

Contraindications: None

Calcium

Add calcium if you are in trouble leaning toward mania.

Calcium

RDA: 1 g (1,000 mg) daily

Recommended dose (in balance): 1 g daily

Recommended dose (in trouble): 1–2 g daily

Maximum safe level: Unknown

Contraindications: Consult with a doctor before taking calcium if you have a history of kidney stones.

INTERVENTIONS—FOR TIMES OF TROUBLE ONLY

The following supplements are not for daily use over the long term; rather, they are specifically for rebalancing your brain chemistry when you are in trouble. Once your diet is under control and your body in balance, you most likely won't need these supplements. For information on using natural and prescription therapies together, see page 102.

The following sections will cover supplements for Stars in trouble in depression and in mania. Here, we'll start with the nutrients Stars in trouble can take advantage of for mood stabilization in general, no matter what phase they are in.

INTERVENTIONS FOR STARS IN EITHER PHASE

Tryptophan

Tryptophan has a sedative effect that is helpful in treating depression (for a full discussion of depression and tryptophan, see Chapter 3: The Stoic). It can also help quiet the manic patient, and is an excellent sleep aid. The body uses tryptophan to make monoamine neurotransmitters, including serotonin, adrenaline, dopamine, and gamma-aminobutyric acid (GABA). Low

INTERVENTIONS FOR STARS IN TROUBLE (DEPRESSION)

INTERVENTION	DAILY DOSE
Amino Acids	
Tryptophan	1–9 g daily
5-HTP	100 mg 2–3 times a day
Tyrosine	1.5–3 g daily
Phenylalanine	1.5–3 g daily
Herbs	
St. John's wort	300 mg 3 times a day
Ginseng	follow package directions
Minerals	
Cesium	100 mg every 3 months
Zinc	30 mg daily
Lithium aspartate	5–45 mg

INTERVENTIONS FOR STARS IN TROUBLE (MANIA)

INTERVENTION	DAILY DOSE
Amino Acids	
Tryptophan	1–9 g daily
5-HTP	100–300 mg daily
Taurine	1 g daily
Glutamine	500 mg 4 times a day
Herbs	
Ginseng	follow package directions
Kava	100–300 mg daily
Chamomile	3–4 cups of tea daily
Passionflower	1–2 cups at bedtime
Minerals	
Lithium aspartate	5–45 mg

serotonin can cause depression, anxiety, irritability, impatience, impulsivity, abusiveness, short attention span, concentration problems, blocked creativity, lack of focus, scatteredness, a very short fuse, and insomnia—all problems common in the agitated depressed state. In general, tryptophan also helps relieve stress.

Tryptophan

Recommended dose (in trouble): 1,500–9,000 mg daily, in three divided doses.

Maximum safe level: Unknown. Don't exceed 3 grams a day unless you are under a doctor's close supervision. Theoretically, if L-tryptophan raises serotonin too high, serotonin syndrome can result, characterized by confusion, fever, shivering, sweating, diarrhea, muscle spasms, and, very rarely, death.

Contraindications: Don't drive or operate heavy machinery, at least until you develop tolerance and it no longer makes you sleepy.

Studies using tryptophan to treat mania show benefits even in patients ill enough to require hospitalization. One study showed 12 g a day over one week eliminated or cut down on manic symptoms in newly hospitalized patients. Another showed that tryptophan (taken together with pyridoxine [vitamin B6]) performed equally as well as a common prescription drug (also taken with B6) in controlling manic symptoms. Yet another study demonstrated improvement in both manic and borderline manic patients taking tryptophan: When the tryptophan was stopped, the patients relapsed. Another study demonstrated that tryptophan can boost the effectiveness of lithium, though anyone taking lithium should consult with a doctor before trying tryptophan.

The other amino acids in protein will compete with tryptophan, so it is best to take it with carbohydrates and separate from proteins.

5-HTP (5-Hydroxy-Tryptophan)

Studies have shown that 5-HTP can be beneficial in depression. Because of their similarities, 5-HTP ought to work as tryptophan does in mania as well as depression. Studies to date look only at depression, unfortunately, but I recommend it for both on the strength of tryptophan's performance.

5-HTP

Recommended dose (in trouble): 100–200 mg 3 times a day

Maximum safe level: Unknown.

Contraindications: As with L-tryptophan, there is the rare theoretical risk of serotonin syndrome.

Ginseng

Because this herb has calming as well as stimulant effects, Stars in trouble can take it in either manic or depressive phases. Ginseng stimulates the adrenal glands and the "cholinergic" (calming) nervous system. Unlike other stimulants, ginseng doesn't produce nervousness, but rather a feeling of relaxation and well-being. It can also be used as a very mild tranquilizer.

Ginseng

Recommended dose (in trouble): Varies according to the source. Follow package label. (See page 101 for more information.)

Maximum safe level: Unknown

Contraindications: Don't take ginseng if you have anxiety, manic depression, heart palpitations, asthma, or emphysema. Not for use during pregnancy. Do not use it at the same time as caffeine, ephedra, or other stimulants if you have high blood pressure or migraines, or if you are sick.

Lithium

The alkali mineral lithium is frequently prescribed by doctors for patients diagnosed as manic-depressive. The benefits of high doses of lithium carbonate in preventing and treating manic states are clear, but so are the drawbacks. There are many side effects, including nausea, vomiting, tremors, kidney dysfunction, and depression of the thyroid. Lithium is also toxic at doses not much higher than those considered therapeutic.

But low-dose lithium aspartate helps provide the mood-stabilizing benefits of lithium without the side effects, especially when it is used in combination with other nutrients. It is available without a prescription under the brand name Lithate. In the aspartate form, lithium is said to be about ten times more effective than lithium carbonate, so it is possible to give therapeutic doses without risking toxic side effects. Lithium aspartate is available without a prescription, but can be hard to find. You can order it directly from the manufacturer, Bio-Tech Pharmacal at 1-800-345-1199. Tell them Dr. Lesser sent you. I get no commission, but they sure appreciate me!

The body doesn't make lithium, but it is found naturally in our environment because it is a component of the earth's crust, and we get trace amounts in water and food. (Tobacco also contains a good dose of lithium, and some Stars may be unknowingly self-medicating with cigarettes, making it even harder than normal for them to break the addiction.) Lithium aspartate is sold in 5-mg tablets (compared to the 300-mg capsules of lithium carbonate) and has the additional advantage of being organic, while lithium carbonate is an inorganic salt.

Lithium in any form is appropriate for Stars in trouble in either phase. That's particularly important because Stars must be careful with the usual antidepressants, lest they work so well that Stars are pushed into mania. Lithium controls mania by inhibiting the release of the monoamines (including noradrenaline, adrenaline, and dopamine). Lithium also evens out

---

Lithium Aspartate

Recommended dose (in trouble): 5 mg 1–8 times daily as needed

Maximum safe level: Don't take more than 4 doses daily unless you are under a doctor's close supervision.

Contraindications: Taking lithium can result in kidney or cardiovascular disease, dehydration, and salt depletion. Take salt liberally.

blood sugar levels. Whatever the mechanism or mechanisms in operation, lithium changes the cycling of the brain's chemistry to eliminate drastic mood swings.

Lithium carbonate alters sodium transport in nerves, so if you take it, be sure to sprinkle salt liberally on your food.

I rarely prescribe lithium (carbonate) at the usual doses because of the risk of side effects and the need for regular blood tests to monitor levels in the body. I employ only one or two 300-mg lithium carbonate capsules, along with vitamin C (2 grams) to acidify the body and make the lithium more effective in patients unwilling or unable to address their underlying low blood sugar condition. At this level, it is rarely necessary to check blood lithium levels. I prefer to use the low-dose lithium aspartate (three to six 5-mg tablets daily), especially in patients just learning to get their diets under control. For the overexcited Star having trouble sleeping, I use the herbs chamomile and/or passionflower as teas; the mineral sedatives magnesium and zinc; the vitamins inositol (1,500 mg) and vitamin C (500 mg); and the amino acid tryptophan.

And of course I have treated many patients already taking high doses of lithium under another doctor's guidance. After the prescribed nutrients, improved diet, and lifestyle changes I suggest have had a chance to take hold, I often help them lower their dose of lithium. Use lithium aspartate only under a doctor's supervision.

Natural Sources of Lithium

Tobacco

Sugarcane

Seaweed

French mineral waters such as Lithee, Apollinaire, Vicy, and Perrier

INTERVENTIONS FOR STARS IN THE DEPRESSION PHASE

As for what works for Stars in trouble in depression, the list looks much like what is recommended for Stoics (see Chapter 3: The Stoic for further information on these supplements).

Zinc

In addition to balancing excessively high copper during depression (or when zinc is deficient in relation to normal copper levels), zinc has a sedating effect that makes it good for calming mania. Copper is also frequently

---

Zinc

RDA: 15 mg

Recommended Dose (in balance): 30 mg daily

Recommended Dose (in trouble): 80–160 mg daily for a few weeks at a time, in manic crisis.

Maximum safe level: Unknown. One boy who consumed 12,000 mg (12 grams) zinc overslept for four days, fell asleep frequently through the day, wrote in an illegible scrawl, staggered when he walked. Completely recovered by sixth day; no permanent harm.

Contraindications: Coma

---

high in mania, and zinc low. In those cases, just enough zinc to balance the copper may help ease mania. But large doses of zinc are calming, whatever the copper level. Excessive blood zinc can cause a copper and iron deficiency anemia, though, so it is best to use zinc only as a therapeutic weapon during mania or to correct an imbalance. Everyone needs zinc for mental calmness and well-being, balanced with a normal amount of copper for alertness and attentiveness.

Tyrosine

Many people do not seem to respond to tyrosine, but for those who do, it can be a powerful choice. Tyrosine is an antidepressant because it is used to

> **Tyrosine**
>
> **Recommended dose (in trouble):** 1.5–3 g daily
>
> **Maximum safe level:** Unknown
>
> **Contraindications:** Do not take tyrosine with MAOIs. If you are taking a prescription drug for depression, discuss it with your doctor before you start taking tyrosine. Do not take it if you have active cancer.

make adrenaline, noradrenaline, and dopamine, all of which regulate mood. It is particularly helpful for people with low levels of thyroid hormone.

Phenylalanine

This amino acid, which the body converts into tyrosine, is a stimulant and a fast-acting antidepressant good for mild (but not severe) cases of depression. Most people respond well to it. You'll have a choice between L-phenylalanine and DL-phenylalanine, and while both can be effective, I recommend the L-form (unless you are also dealing with chronic pain, in which case DL is for you).

In a study of phenylalanine (given together with pyridoxine [vitamin

> **L-Phenylalanine**
>
> **Recommended dose (in trouble):** 1.5–3 g daily. Takes effect about 20 minutes after ingestion. Antidepressant effect appears in 3–6 days.
>
> **Maximum safe level:** 15 g daily (Some people have headaches with 4 g or more.)
>
> **Contraindications:** Don't take phenylalanine with MAO inhibitors. Don't take if pregnant or nursing, or if you suffer from anxiety attacks, diabetes, high blood pressure, phenylketonuria (PKU), Wilson's disease, or skin cancer. Not appropriate for children.

B6]), most depressed patients showed immediate improvement. A quarter recovered completely. The results were even stronger in bipolar patients (manic depression) than in those with unipolar depression.

DL-Phenylalanine (for pain, i.e., migraines)

Recommended dose (in trouble): 500 mg daily three times a day for one week, then once daily

Maximum Safe Level: Unknown

Contraindications: Don't take phenylalanine with MAO inhibitors. Don't take if pregnant or nursing, or if you suffer from anxiety attacks, diabetes, high blood pressure, phenylketonuria (PKU), Wilson's disease or active cancer. Not appropriate for children.

St. John's Wort (Hypericum)

Widely used in Europe for years to treat mild to moderate depression, this herb is very useful as an antidepressant and sedative. It is the most widely

---

St. John's Wort

Recommended dose (in trouble): 300 mg 3 times a day

Contraindications: Do not take St. John's wort with MAO inhibitors (or for four weeks after stopping them); coumidin; digoxin; protease inhibitors; indinavir (for HIV); cyclosporine (for cancer); or photosensitizing drugs, including tetracycline. Do not take it while on drugs following a transplant. Not for pregnant or nursing women. Can speed up the breakdown of (interfering with the effectiveness of) prescription medication, including blood thinners, cholesterol-lowering medications, seizure medications, cancer medications, drugs used to fight HIV, drugs that prevent organ transplant rejection, and birth control pills.

studied natural antidepressant and has been proven to match (and sometimes surpass) the results of prescription drugs. Some people feel the effects of St. John's wort immediately, and for some people it takes up to six weeks (just as with the prescription antidepressants). If you are using a prescription treatment, do not switch to St. John's wort except under the supervision of your doctor.

Stars must take special care with St. John's wort, as the herb can act as a stimulant, working synergistically with mood. Stars should not take it on its own during a manic phase. However, St. John's wort works well in conjunction with lithium. That combination is only for use under the close supervision of a medical professional.

Cesium

Many of my mild to moderately depressed patients have had success with cesium.

Cesium

Recommended dose (in trouble): 100 mg once every 3 months or up to 400 mg every day (only under the supervision of a physician)

Contraindications: This mineral is not for women of childbearing age; may increase anxiety.

INTERVENTIONS FOR THE STAR IN THE MANIC PHASE

In bipolar disorders, there are also a host of useful treatments for the manic component. The most effective ones follow.

Taurine

The inhibitory amino acid taurine is found throughout mammalian brains. The human body uses it for the digestion of fats and fat-soluble vitamins, and to make proper use of sodium, calcium, and magnesium. It has a calming effect on the nervous system (including the brain), so a deficiency can cause hyperactivity, anxiety, and poor general brain function.

Taurine is a *non*-essential amino acid because, unlike the essential ones, it can be manufactured in the body from the amino acids methionine and cysteine, when assisted by pyridoxine (vitamin B6). It has an inhibitory calming effect on the nervous system, stimulating the most potent of all the inhibitory neurotransmitters (including GABA).

Women in particular need to make sure that they take in enough taurine, since estrogen depresses formation of taurine in the liver. Women using supplemental estrogen need even more.

Alcohol causes the excretion of taurine in urine and interferes with the body's ability to use what it has properly. That's particularly a problem in hypoglycemia, which increases the need for taurine. Diabetes increases the need for taurine, as it has an influence on blood sugar levels similar to that of insulin. (If you use insulin and begin taking taurine, you should talk to your doctor about the possibility of lowering your insulin dose.)

Taurine is present in animal, not vegetable, proteins, so vegetarians need to be careful to get enough.

For the Star in trouble who is in an overexcited manic phase, I use a series of varying doses of taurine (see below), supported by 100 mg zinc sul-

---

Taurine

Recommended dose (in balance): 50 mg daily

Recommended dose (in trouble): 1,000 mg the first day, 500 mg the second day, 200 mg the third day, 150 mg the fourth day, 100 mg the fifth day, 50 mg the sixth day—then rest for two weeks and repeat the six-day cycle.

Maximum safe level: Unknown. Up to 6 g daily has been used safely.

Contraindications: Since it can be irritating to digestive tract, don't use taurine if you have an ulcer. Nausea sometimes occurs with high doses (above 10 grams).

fate (which also has a sedating effect on the brain), 100 mg vitamin B6, and 2,000 mg glutamine (to make the calming amino acid GABA).

Glutamine

The amino acid glutamine, together with pyridoxine (vitamin B6), produces GABA (a natural tranquilizer) in the brain. See Chapter 3: The Stoic for details.

L-Glutamine

Recommended dose (in trouble): 500 mg four times a day

Maximum safe level: Unknown; studies have used up to 60 g without toxicity

Contraindications: None

Kava

Although this herb is stimulating in small amounts, larger amounts (as in the doses recommended here) are sedating. Kava induces calm feelings and eases muscle tension. It sharpens the mind and quiets your internal dialogue. See Chapter 4: The Guardian for details.

Kava

Recommended dose: 1 to 3 sprays a day of liquid (60 mg of 30 percent kavalactones per spray); or in powder or capsules, 100 mg of 70 percent kavalactones daily

Maximum safe level: Unknown

Contraindications: Kava can exacerbate Parkinson's disease. Do not take it with alcohol; barbiturates, benzodiazepines, or any major tranquilizer; anticoagulants or antiplatelet agents (including aspirin); antipsychotics; drugs for treating Parkinson's disease; or drugs that depress the central nervous system.

Chamomile

Chamomile is a mildly sedative, calming, and relaxing herb. See Chapter 4: The Guardian for more information.

Chamomile

Recommended dose: 3–4 cups of tea daily

Maximum safe level: Unknown

Contraindications: If you are allergic to ragweed, chrysanthemums, and other daisies, you may want to avoid chamomile, which is in the same family. (You won't necessarily be sensitive to it, though, so it may be worth a try.)

Passionflower

This sedative herb is mildly calming and reduces restlessness.

Passionflower

Recommended dose: 4–8 g (dry herb, or taken as tea) daily; or extract standardized to 1.2 percent apigenin and .5 percent essential oils; or 300–450 mg of the dry powdered extract (2.6 percent flavonoids)

Maximum safe level: Unknown

Contraindications: Unknown

Mind/Body and Lifestyle Changes

For most types, I recommend learning a thing or two from some of the other types with complementary strengths, especially those next to or across from yours on the pie chart (p. 28). But Stars are already experienced with both an outer-directed and an inner-directed style and the benefits that come from drawing on the full spectrum. What Stars often need to improve is the communication between the introspective and extroverted sides of their personality. Stars can benefit from learning how to get the best of both worlds and make them work together.

Stars will benefit most from calming practices like yoga, meditation, religious study, or other spiritual practices. Stars tend to be overly active and outer-directed, and anything centering and inner-directed can provide a useful counterbalance. Behavior reflects brain chemistry—but brain chemistry also reflects behavior. As a Star, if you act nervous and tense all the time, those are the messages your neurotransmitters will be carrying. If you practice being tranquil, the message will be quite different. For a manic person needing to slow down, this can be a chicken-or-egg situation. So I say, why not take advantage of both: good nutrition to "slow" overactive brain chemistry and actions, while those slower actions work to stabilize your brain chemistry.

Deep breathing exercises can be perfect for manic Stars or anyone who is feeling manic or anxious. Sit or stand straight and still in a silent environment, where the air is as fresh and clean as possible. Let your arms rest at your side and close your mouth so you are breathing only through your nostrils. (If you can't breathe through both nostrils, this most likely means you have a food allergy or cold. Food allergies themselves can, cause bipolar mood swings.) Inhale slowly and steadily for seven seconds. Try to make a sound with your breathing as the air enters your nostrils. Breathe as deeply as you can, expanding your lungs down into your stomach and the small of the back. Hold the air in for a count of two seconds, then exhale slowly and steadily through the nose for seven seconds, as fully as you can, to get rid of all the stale and musty air that's been hanging around in your lungs. Repeat this cycle for ten or twelve breaths, two or three times a day, or whenever you are anxious. It's remarkable how many of my anxious and overexcited patients find this is all they need to calm down. Not only is deep breathing a lot safer than tranquilizer drugs, and less expensive even than vitamins, but oxygen is our most vital and frequently lacking nutrient.

TALK THERAPY

The protective, nurturing environment cultivated in insight psychotherapy (see page 108 in Chapter 3: The Stoic) can help Stars accommodate to the inevitable vicissitudes of their condition. But insight psychotherapy requires calm, sober reasoning; concentration; clear thinking (even on sensitive topics); and a willingness to look at your own faults and be critical of yourself, which is often not possible for a Star in a manic phase. Stars in the "up" parts of the cycle usually don't even perceive a need for help or a reason for change.

However, if a Star in trouble has swung low rather than high, insight psychotherapy might be productive. If there's anything good about depression, it is that reason usually is maintained. Doctors and counselors often prefer working with Stars in this part of the cycle because depressed Stars can think clearly and have insight into themselves (a prerequisite, naturally, for insight therapy).

In my practice, I do a unique kind of insight therapy, based not so much on the psychological but the physiological. Helping someone make the connection between their addictions and their behavior (as with the patient with the caffeine problem I described earlier) or their diet and their moods (as with Fred and his diet) will give the patient welcome control over his or her mood swings.

That still fits the general theory in insight psychotherapy that figuring out what your problems are and what causes them is the key to undoing them. In this tradition, a therapist would never tell you what to do, but would only guide you on your own internal exploration. Supportive therapy, on the other hand, is designed to help you figure out what to do, with the therapist lending the benefit of another mind devoted to the subject. In the rare case when a manic Star seeks help, supportive therapy may be the most likely to work. In this case, a therapist may make suggestions on how to reign in out-of-control emotions and behavior and prevent recurrences of mania. For example, simply telling a manic Star to get some sleep and eat regular meals may be very supportive. Without this intervention, a Star can be so caught in a web of mental excitement that he can't see the basics, like the need for rest and refueling. In depression severe enough to be paralyzing, supportive therapy may also be more appropriate than insight.

As discussed in Chapter 3: The Stoic, depression is usually set off by a loss, and identifying the loss and helping the patient deal with it are major goals of therapy. For example, Sarah (in the first chapter) was thrown out of balance emotionally by her repeated miscarriages. In my own case, my two major quiet cycles were set off by losses, the first after the death of my parents and the second after my house burned down.

Manic phases, on the other hand, are linked not directly to loss, but to *gain*. Too much gain makes Stars in trouble overly optimistic, overproud, and overconfident. Mania is basically the period before a loss happens. Stars are destined to fall because they have climbed too high, and a loss is bound to happen eventually.

Whether you are using insight or supportive therapy—or whether you are getting therapy at all—the most important thing for Stars to do in the psychological realm is to get in touch with the positive aspects of their type. The negatives often take precedence—they are what make us seek help, after all. But our types are deeply embedded in us, and we shouldn't be aiming to get rid of our natural tendencies. Rather, our goal must be to make the most of our innate abilities and talents and to ensure a stable balance among all our polarities so our weak points are protected and our strengths take the lead.

7

The Dreamer

Of all the profiles, the Dreamer is the rarest (probably 1 percent of the population), most complex, and least understood. When Dreamers are able to actualize their total potential, they are the visionaries who bring their extraordinary fantasies to fruition. But they are vulnerable to losing themselves in their dreams and withdrawing into their own world. Among psychiatrists, the label of choice for this profile is schizoid. Dreamers in trouble get diagnosed as having borderline personality disorder or, in extreme cases, schizophrenia.

Dreamers are deeply concerned about their spiritual lives, to the point where they frequently neglect their physical and material well-being. They give away money when they don't have enough themselves. They forget to turn off the burner after the water has boiled. They "let themselves go"—sometimes forgoing personal grooming because they just can't be bothered and, in the extremes of the type in trouble, ignoring even basic hygiene. They forget to eat, which can create malnutrition of the brain, setting the stage for the extreme behavior of the Dreamer in trouble. As far as the material world goes, Dreamers embrace the "It's all small stuff" part of *Don't Sweat the Small Stuff.*

Many of the great religious leaders throughout history have been Dreamers. They often have an intense, intimate, personal relationship with their God. Dreamers are open to levels of reality most of us close off. Martin Luther, the founder of Protestantism, for example, heard voices. When some Dreamers are chemically out of balance, they believe that they *are* God. Dreamers are by no means limited to the religious sphere—Sir Isaac Newton, the father of modern physics, reportedly heard voices as well.

Dreamers are introspective, inner-directed, and often absorbed in their internal life. They appreciate and sometimes crave solitude. Others often perceive them to be alienated, asocial loners, or even antisocial eccentrics.

Dreamers are compassionate and empathetic, and frequently want to act accordingly, serving others and being helpful whenever possible. They are highly sensitive to their environment and easily influenced by their own base instincts as well as outside factors. They are exquisitely tuned in to what others think and do, but they often jump to conclusions, misunderstanding or misinterpreting what they observe. To a Dreamer in trouble, even an offhand remark or well-intentioned comment can become a serious insult. This reveals one of the great paradoxes of the Dreamer: On the one hand, they can be so assured it is impossible to deter the pursuit of their passion. On the other hand, but they often lack self-confidence of the most basic sort.

Generally highly intelligent and holding lofty moral standards, Dreamers are nonetheless humble and are generally sweet, gentle, and pleasant to be around. But they are also quick to anger and then are torn over their intense desire to avoid conflict. That tension is often what drives Dreamers in trouble too far into a dreamworld, causing them to disconnect with reality.

Dreamers tend to be brighter and more competent than the rest of us—as long as they don't become imbalanced. Properly nourished, they are some of the most advanced people on the planet, and certainly the smartest people likely to come into my office. (Usually, they are there because someone else can't understand them.) Some of the most influential people in history have been Dreamers, because they can conceive of ideas beyond most people's capability. Their singleness of vision, unwavering commitment, and willingness to self-sacrifice bring those ideas to fruition. Dreamers march to the beat of a different drummer, so even when they are not in trouble, there's a real risk they'll be misunderstood. After all, visionaries are rarely understood at the beginning of their work.

I'll give you just one example of a Dreamer that illustrates the religious obsession that often surfaces in Dreamers in trouble. This poor and illiterate person was barely in her teens when she began to hear voices no one else heard. Saints sent by God were talking to her on a regular basis. Following their commands, she cut off her long hair, dressed in men's clothes, and heavily armed herself. She then announced her intention to overthrow the government and began seeking recruits for her divine mission.

This Dreamer—Joan of Arc—was burned at the stake for heresy when she was just nineteen years old because she wouldn't renounce her "voices." Despite this unhappy ending, her heroism and passionate faith stand as reminders of the potential greatness within all Dreamers. Starting with noth-

Type	General Traits	Beneficial Aspects	Harmful Aspects	Vulnerabilities
Dreamers	Visionary	Have high moral	Are easily slighted.	Dreamers in
	Humble	standards.	Are ill at ease socially.	trouble tend
	Spiritual	Don't care about	Have a weak sense	toward border-
	Sensitive	material things.	of self.	line personality
	Gentle	March to the beat of a	Are internal.	disorder and,
	Introspective	different drummer.	Feel alienated and	in the most
	Solitary	Can count Vincent	lonely.	extreme cases,
	Cerebral	van Gogh as one of	Feel unappreciated	schizophrenia.
	Shy	their own.	or unrecognized.	
	Eccentric		Can't handle (or even	
			recognize) anger.	
			Are misunderstood,	
			vulnerable, and	
			withdrawn.	
			Are easily influenced.	
			Lack self-confidence.	
			Avoid conflict at all	
			costs.	
			Go to extremes.	

ing more than the force of her vision, Joan of Arc assembled an army, led them into battle, scored a stunning upset victory, and crowned a new king. If she were alive today, the bizarre symptoms she displayed might get her dosed up with heavy-duty tranquilizers or institutionalized. She'd most likely be no better understood now than she was in her own time, which should teach all of us a lesson: How are we treating the unrecognized "saints" among us now?

Dreamer Profile: Vincent van Gogh

If you were assigned the "pro" side of a debate on "Madness and Genius," you might well have Vincent van Gogh on the top of your list of examples. After all, this is the man almost as famous for cutting off his ear as for his painting "The Starry Night."

Like so many Dreamers, van Gogh's genius (if not his "madness") was unrecognized in his own time—he hadn't sold a single painting before he died. His life story provides a reasonably complete checklist of schizophrenic symptoms. But there's good evidence that poor nutrition was to blame for many of his troubles. And though he sometimes claimed his illness improved or even made possible his work—a popular "mad genius" theory—I wonder what marvels might have been possible had he been able to properly balance his brain chemistry.

Van Gogh's own words paint a clear picture of exactly what he wrestled with. His many and voluminous letters to his brother, collected and published as *Dear Theo: The Autobiography of Vincent van Gogh*, shed much light on the causes and effects of his condition.

In his letters, van Gogh had a lot to say on poverty, probably because it was such an overwhelming daily reality for him. He rarely worked and, like many Dreamers in trouble, was dependent on

(continued)

Dreamer Profile: Vincent van Gogh *(continued)*

others for, literally, his daily bread. For lack of money, van Gogh constantly wanted for even the basic raw materials of his art. He was so desperate it often came down to the grimmest of choices: "The expenses of living, wherever it may be, are always a least 100 francs a month; if one has less, it means want, either physically or of the necessary materials and tools." (He was by no means "living large"—100 francs is the equivalent of about $14.50 today.)

Van Gogh often literally starved himself for his work. "I have had continually to choose between fasting and working alas, insofar as possible I've chosen the former," he wrote.

He was quite literally right about the trade-offs he was making between food and supplies, of course, but also in the connection between lack of food and nutrition and mental as well as physical health. It is a wonder he had the wherewithal to have that insight into himself, when you consider what he was subsisting on. As reported to his brother, "My chief food is dry bread and some potatoes and chestnuts . . . taking now and then a somewhat better meal in a restaurant whenever I can afford it will help set me right again." Again, both the disease and the cure—eating well and regularly—were clear, if unattainable, to van Gogh.

The poor money skills, irregular employment, financial dependence on others, and neglect of physical needs are all common in Dreamers in trouble. Van Gogh's letters trace many other typical sticking points. For example, he confesses, "I have often neglected my appearance; this I admit, and I admit that it is shocking," and blames poverty, discouragement, and *the need to assure solitude.* Even in the roughest times, van Gogh had extraordinary insight into himself. I find it particularly interesting what lengths Dreamers will go to in order to be able to inhabit their own world, on their own.

(continued)

Dreamer Profile: Vincent van Gogh *(continued)*

Like many Dreamers, even those closest to him didn't begin to fathom him: "Father and mother are very good at heart, but have little understanding of our inward feelings. . . . They are very good to me and kinder than ever. But I should rather they could understand more my thoughts and opinions about many things."

On the other hand, van Gogh could not have been easy to relate to. Many Dreamers struggle with interpersonal relationships, and true to form, van Gogh describes bitter falling-outs with various friends. He himself says, "I should see the future less darkly if I were less awkward in dealing with people."

Many times van Gogh returns to the subjects of God, morality, and conscience. As is typical of Dreamers, these subjects were of the utmost importance to him.

Several different times he catalogs his physical ailments. During bouts of paranoia, he writes of his fears, including that people wanted to poison him, that a petition was circulating describing him as not fit to be at liberty, and that the management of the hospital he was in was able, clever, and powerful, and so somehow sinister.

I'm sure van Gogh spoke for all misunderstood Dreamers in trouble when he wrote, "I cannot believe, Theo, that I could be such a monster of impudence and impoliteness as to deserve to be cut off from society." But I'm not sure society has improved tolerance, empathy, or treatment very much in the intervening century or so.

Had he been a well-nourished Dreamer, with a rich inner life and a burning ambition for expression unlike anything the world had yet known, I think van Gogh would have had a longer and even more productive and revolutionary career. Great Dreamers like Joan

(continued)

Dreamer Profile: Vincent van Gogh *(continued)*

of Arc show what is possible when one is capable of fully engaging in the world—albeit in true Dreamer fashion. Van Gogh was too often in extremes for us to believe that, despite his enormous contribution, he achieved all he might have. That's a tremendous loss to the world, and he paid the price in personal satisfaction as well.

Van Gogh once summed up his vision—and the fact that he did so without any actual evidence that his work would endure, much less become internationally treasured masterpieces, demonstrated the strength of the Dreamer's blind faith. I'll let him have the last words, as they can serve as a motto for any Dreamer: "Our work remains, but we do not, and the principal thing is to create."

Accentuate the Positive

Of all the profiles, Dreamers are probably most in need of reclaiming the positive aspects of their type. In the popular imagination, and even to most doctors and many Dreamers themselves, this type is associated with the extremes of trouble: delusions, hallucinations, inappropriate affect, autistic behavior, extreme withdrawal, and disordered thinking. The negative label and stereotypic assumptions are so powerful—and, granted, the behavior often so confounding to the rest of us—that the larger picture, and especially the plusses, is missing.

Their own lack of self-confidence can block Dreamers' view of the benefits, an effect greatly compounded by others' misperceptions reflected back at them. The irony is twofold: Dreamers, by rights, should hold their heads highest of all. But they are also most likely to be treated shabbily by the world. That's definitely true when they are out of balance, but it even holds when they are well nourished, in balance, and just being their own unique Dreamer selves. It isn't easy being misunderstood.

It is because this profile is so poorly understood, by society at large and even within the medical community and by Dreamers themselves, that I have spent so much time describing many of the typical personality traits above. More than any other profile, what the person is like is as useful as what his or her blood chemistry is like in determining where he or she fits in this typology.

Dreamer Subtypes

No blood chemistry marker is typical of the biochemical profile of the Dreamer. The only common ground is that whatever the results, they are usually extreme. One Dreamer may be very high on a particular marker, while the next one may be quite low.

To help make sense of the wide range of results in blood chemistry markers in Dreamers, we're going to look at four subcategories: Stoic Dreamers, Star Dreamers, Warrior Dreamers, and Borderline Dreamers. As you might guess, each of the first three kinds of Dreamers shares many of the characteristics of the profiles they are named after, as well as many of the blood chemistry markers. Borderline Dreamers I'll explain below.

The subtypes apply only to Dreamers in trouble. In balance, those tendencies do not emerge.

For Dreamers in trouble, diagnosis is the hard part. Once it is done, treatment is simpler, requiring straightforward matching of symptoms, signs, markers, and solutions. Understanding yourself as a Dreamer, and recognizing your subtype, will lead you directly to the changes you need to make to avoid the pitfalls of your profile. Or, if you are out of balance, it will give you leads as to what testing and treatment will be most helpful.

As we look at each subtype here, we will examine the blood chemistry markers most often found in that subtype.

STOIC DREAMERS

Stoic Dreamers tend to have a fast metabolism, be sensitive to pain, have trouble sleeping, experience seasonal allergies, and experience sexual orgasm quickly.

Stoic Dreamers in trouble are usually depressed and might have phobias, obsessions, or compulsions. They appear somber and sober, and they see their situation realistically. At the extremes, this is the type with the most real risk of suicide.

Stoic Dreamers in trouble typically have high blood histamine and/or low blood serotonin, just like Stoics in trouble. Serum copper levels are usually normal. Many also have flat curve hypoglycemia (again like Stoics), and some have low thyroid hormone. About 20 percent of Dreamers have high histamine, and about 10 percent have low serotonin.

STAR DREAMERS

Star Dreamers in trouble often have low histamine and/or high serotonin—just like Stars in trouble in the manic phase. They often suffer from the same mania characterized by an elated, excited state, grandiosity, and sometimes even auditory hallucinations (voices) and delusions. They usually have a slow metabolism. They also have a low basophil count and high copper levels.

Star Dreamers with low histamine rarely suffer from colds or allergy. About 15 percent of Dreamers have high serotonin, and about 20 percent have low histamine.

WARRIOR DREAMERS

Warrior Dreamers in trouble often have excessively high copper levels (and low zinc). Too much copper can produce schizophrenic symptoms, including serious changes in personality and thought processes, and especially paranoia. One study showed that about 20 percent of schizophrenia patients had high copper levels, and another found high copper to be particularly associated with depression, paranoia, and hallucinations in schizophrenic people. One dramatic example of the connection between copper and schizophrenia can be found in Wilson's disease. The hallmark of the condition is the body's storage of too much copper, and it often first shows up as schizophrenic symptoms. Similarly, so called "dialysis dementia" is thought to be attributable to excess copper.

As always, low zinc goes hand in hand with high copper when it comes to causing problems, as it is the ratio between the two that is of the utmost importance. Zinc deficiency can cause schizophrenic symptoms. One study found that people with schizophrenic symptoms had zinc levels that were half that of those in a control group. Another study found low zinc in 11 percent of schizophrenic patients. Zinc deficiency has been associated with depression, as we saw in Chapter 3: The Stoic, and also with apathy, lethargy, irritability, and—of particular note for Dreamers in general, and Warrior Dreamers in particular—paranoia.

Warrior Dreamers may also have high levels of thyroid hormone. This is the more common type of hormonal imbalance in Dreamers and is often associated with paranoia. A thyroid panel is an important blood chemistry marker, especially for Warrior Dreamers, and should include a highly sensitive test for thyroid-stimulating hormone (TSH), the thyroid hormones T_3 and T_4, and anti-thyroid antibodies.

Like Warriors in trouble, Warrior Dreamers in trouble can be aggressive and even psychopathic. In Warrior Dreamers, that state is almost always a defensive stance, often in reaction to imagined insults or enemies. They are much less likely than Warriors to turn aggressive proactively.

BORDERLINE DREAMERS

Borderline Dreamers are so called not only because they are on the edges of the category but also because when they are in trouble the symptoms they show are those of borderline personality disorder more than schizophrenic symptoms. Though it is surely oversimplifying matters, for our purposes we can think of borderline personality disorder as a sort of mild form of simple schizophrenia. Borderline Dreamers are less likely to have significant results on any of the biochemical markers. They may well have normal levels of all the usual suspects. In that case, personality characteristics are the best way to identify if you are in this subtype.

The most distinguishing features of borderline personality disorder are impulsivity, intense but unstable relationships with other people—often fluctuating rapidly from high-esteem to complete scorn (and back again)—and equally quick-changing shifts in moods and emotions. Borderline Dreamers tend to have rather nebulous personalities, without much edge to them. They can seem rather "blah," as if nothing much is going on with them, no matter what the internal realities are. A Borderline Dreamer, for example, could be a C-student the teachers never pay much attention to but who has stellar IQ scores buried somewhere in her records.

If Borderline Dreamers have "disperceptions" at all, they will be very mild, nothing that will seriously interfere with daily life. I had one patient, for example, who would hear a "fiery jet" no one else heard when he had angry or hateful thoughts—but had no other significant symptoms.

Cases in Point

CRAIG

Although I've just laid out some of the most common Dreamer subtypes, I don't want to lose sight of the fact that Dreamers have more variability than any other profile. To that end, before we get to the dietary guidelines, supplements, and mind/body strategies that behoove Dreamers, let me introduce you to "Craig," who doesn't fit neatly into any of the subtypes above. He had high histamine and was depressed like a Stoic Dreamer in trouble, but his serotonin was at the high end of normal—high enough to impart a manicky quality to some of his behavior, like a Star Dreamer. He had high copper like a Warrior Dreamer, and he was also hypoglycemic.

In the middle of his high-school career, Craig's grades took a nosedive, particularly in math. He started getting in trouble at school more and more frequently, though he'd always been basically well-behaved up to this point, and his attendance became erratic. He was angry all the time and managed to aggravate just about everyone he came into contact with. He spent long periods of time in his room with the door closed.

At first it seemed like garden-variety adolescent rebellion, but his family was becoming increasingly annoyed and disturbed by his strange and aggressive behavior. When they began to hear odd vocalizations and unintelligible sounds—loud enough to be heard

(continued)

Cases in Point *(continued)*

throughout the house—through that closed door to his room, they became truly concerned for him. That's when he landed in my office.

He told me he'd been feeling out of touch with reality for about a year. He felt depressed, angry, and alienated. He couldn't concentrate. He wasn't any happier about how things were going than the rest of his family, and he was eager to make changes.

Aside from the lab results mentioned above, his body chemistry was normal.

He had white spots on his fingernails, which are a sign of zinc deficiency—or, in this case, relative zinc deficiency. His zinc levels technically fell within the range of normal, but up against his extremely high copper level, the ratio was wildly out of balance. I explained that lack of zinc and too much copper was probably what was making him angry, reclusive, and even paranoid and potentially violent, and I prescribed zinc and manganese supplements. Within three months, his copper to zinc ratio was healthy again.

High copper alone can cause hypoglycemia, and tests confirmed that Craig's blood sugar levels were out of control, so he began following a diet with frequent meals, limited sugars, and simple carbohydrates consisting of whole, natural, unrefined foods. I told him to be sure to get plenty of beans, eggs, milk, and the "smelly" vegetables like garlic, onion, chives, radishes, and asparagus because the sulfur in those foods would help get rid of any heavy metals in his system—copper being almost a heavy metal. Repeat testing confirmed what his mood was already telling us: His hypoglycemia was under control. His serotonin level also moved more solidly into the middle of normal.

To lower his histamine levels, Craig took calcium and methio-

(continued)

Cases in Point *(continued)*

nine. (Methionine in very large doses can cause psychosis, so some-times it is recommended that Dreamers in trouble not use it. I be-lieve it is still helpful and safe and simply tell my patients to stop taking it once the histamine is lowered and the depression lifts.) A follow-up test four months later showed his levels were down, but still too high. I suspected the B-complex vitamin he was taking, with the histamine-raisers niacin, folic acid, and cobalamin (vita-min B12) in it, was to blame, though ordinarily it isn't enough to outweigh the calcium-methionine combination. A high-protein diet, too, can raise histamine. So I had him cut back a bit on pro-tein, without going back to simple carbohydrates or sugars, and add a dimethylglycine supplement (sometimes known as vitamin B15). This vitamin lowers histamine and boosts energy levels. I've used a similar treatment plan to help other patients overcome their need for tranquilizers.

I never did another histamine test on Craig, as we didn't need lab tests to show us how much he'd improved—the real, live boy in front of me told me all I needed to know. His grades climbed. The noises stopped. His friends came around again. He left his room. He went to all his classes. In short, his life resumed its earlier, far nicer course—a normal, adolescent life. I think of Craig as a "future Dreamer in trouble"—identified and treated early enough that he should be able to access the positive aspects of the profile through-out his life, while staying biochemically balanced enough to avoid the potential downsides.

A seemingly contradictory bunch of test results and observa-tions, like those I started with in Craig's case, makes diagnosis more complicated. But fortunately natural medical solutions will still bring relief, though it takes a bit more work to match up the ap-

(continued)

Cases in Point *(continued)*

propriate treatments with the range of symptoms and findings. If you take no other point away from this story, let it be a reminder that while finding yourself within a particular profile or subtype is useful, we are all truly amalgams of different types, with one profile predominating. We can all learn something for every profile, including effective treatments for our own unique group of symptoms and lab results.

ESTHER

Consider what happened to Esther. Her father died when she was sixteen, and at the funeral service, she thought she saw a bright light behind the priest. To her, it was a comforting vision, like a promise she would see her father again, a sign that there's a whole world out there we can't yet understand. But when she told all this to her family and the priest, they became alarmed that she was seeing things. That set off a negative spiral of misunderstanding, with Esther becoming more and more angry and her family becoming more and more convinced something was wrong with her. By summer, Esther found herself shipped off to a quasi-religious "camp" for troubled teenagers founded on a tough-love premise that hard work was the cure for whatever ailed them.

But doing manual labor twelve hours a day, seven days a week and living with kids with all kinds of problems stressed Esther out further still, and she grew belligerent. She tried to run away from camp and physically threatened some staff members and fellow campers. It was decided that she needed medication, and so she was expelled from camp and sent to a psychiatric hospital where she was put on tranquilizers.

But she was still very angry in the hospital and was often kept

(continued)

Cases in Point *(continued)*

in restraints (wrapped tightly in sheets). She had more visions, though they weren't always as gentle and encouraging as the one at her father's funeral had been. She had many sessions of various types of psychotherapy but never had any real success. Because of her extreme "uncooperativeness," as they say in the psychiatric business, she was eventually sent to a state-run institution for long-term care, where she lived for seven years.

Esther was ultimately discharged, allegedly with some improvement, including increased cooperation, but *coincidentally* just at the time the Reagan administration was cleaning out hospitals nationwide. Even on the heavy-duty tranquilizers she still took, she was paranoid and hearing voices. She was also depressed. She came to see me because she wanted to get off the tranquilizers, or at least get them down to a level where she could do something meaningful with her life. She was still a young woman at this point, but so symptomatic and doped up that there was no way she could hold a job, go to school, or participate in quality relationships.

She was a little bit overweight, which I suspected came from years on low-quality institutional meals. Her soft fingernails told me she hadn't been getting as much protein as she needed. She also smoked like a chimney, drank a lot of alcohol, and was a heavy caffeine user—coffee being the method of choice. She was also hypoglycemic.

As she learned about the appropriate diet, I also advised her to cut back on coffee, which she did. She cut out simple sugars, replacing those foods with healthier, whole complex carbohydrates. She began to feel better and stronger, which prompted her to stop drinking coffee and alcohol completely and to quit smoking. That allowed her to cut down on her tranquilizers, and within six months,

(continued)

Cases in Point *(continued)*

she was down to less than half the dose she had started on. Over the next six months, she was able to cut the dose in half again. Two months later she was off the daily drugs altogether, though she'd use a very small dose every once in a while in times of great stress.

Her diet wasn't perfect—she still had birthday cake, champagne toasts at weddings, and other occasional treats. The world is set up like that, and it is difficult if not impossible to avoid. I'm not sure it would even be healthy to deny yourself all those foods forever because of the social value they hold. But the many changes she made got her chemistry into balance, and she was like a new woman. She no longer heard voices or had visions. The thoughtful and philosophical parts of her personality began to dominate, rather than the negative. Her true nature—gentle and humble—resurfaced.

Esther was one of my patients for whom talk therapy was helpful. Without chemical imbalances creating out-of-control moods and keeping her angry all the time, she could recognize her anger for what it was: the core hurt she felt at never having been understood. She had simply seen a light no one else had. *She* hadn't freaked out when she saw that vision behind the priest. But the people around her, the ones who loved and cared for her and were supposed to know her best, did freak out. It was tough information for her to process, but Esther slowly sorted herself out and moved forward with her reclaimed life.

She went to technical school and got a well-paying job in her field when she finished. She learned to make—and keep—friends, and eventually met and married a man who *did* understand her. She is a success story.

(continued)

Cases in Point *(continued)*

But I think of her case together with Craig's because I believe the right response early in her life (as in Craig's case) could have saved Esther years of pain. On the flip side, Craig could have been an Esther. Or worse, Craig could have been Esther in the life she would have lived if no one had come up with something better than tranquilizers to help her. We can all begin by carefully considering our judgments of others, backed by what we've learned about the positive aspects of each profile. Learning to look at ourselves is the first step, but our work is not done until we also use it to look at others.

Dietary Guidelines

To live the Dreamers' dream—a balanced, earth-bound life allowing for a visionary's work—proper diet is essential. It will allow you to maximize the positive aspects of your type and minimize the potential negatives. It provides the necessary foundation for the supplements recommended later in this chapter to do their work, and it facilitates the success of any mind/body strategies you choose as well.

Less than optimal brain nutrition can be a problem for every one of us, but Dreamers are particularly likely to be malnourished. First, most Dreamers have a casual attitude toward their physical health and so are less likely to be concerned about nutrition. Second, their brains are the most sensitive of any of the types and need even better nutrition than the rest of us to function at their peak. As a result, Dreamers must be more strict with their diets, even when in balance, than some of the other types. Because of their finely tuned nervous systems, Dreamers must stick closely to their diet at all times.

Almost all Dreamers in trouble—about 85 percent by my experience—have malnourished brains, with shortages of micronutrients (vitamins and minerals) as well as macronutrients (proteins and fats). About two-thirds of Dreamers have hypoglycemia. Just eating healthfully in accordance with their profile can make a world of difference.

Of all the profiles, Dreamers tend to have the worst overall diets, with sugar being the biggest troublemaker. Many Dreamers are easy pushovers for junk food. It is just one of the ways they are sensitive to their environment—if they want to eat, they eat what's in front of them (which, in this society, is likely to be heavily refined) or whatever they want at the moment, without regard to how it affects the body. Or, they can be so lost in another world (in trouble) or just be focused so exclusively on spiritual matters that they pay no attention to what they eat. They are also vulnerable to addictions, of which addiction to sugar is most common. And Dreamers in trouble suffer terribly. The torment they go through, both real and imagined, can be severe, so it is no wonder they feel entitled to a bit of immediate gratification. Here again, a vicious cycle occurs—being malnourished creates a Dreamer in trouble; and a Dreamer in trouble makes poor choices about food, creating malnutrition.

In summary, Dreamers need a high-protein diet that is moderate in fat and low in animal fat in particular. It must also be low in sugar and simple carbohydrates. We'll get to the specific food choices Dreamers should make in a moment.

Many Dreamers are vegetarians (some for spiritual reasons, and some simply because of a lack of affinity for meat). A vegetarian diet rich in non-meat protein and low in simple carbohydrates and sugars can be supportive—but it is more difficult to arrange and maintain. This may be more of a challenge than some Dreamers are up to when they are in trouble, or more than they simply want to deal with in a worldly plane when they are not. However, most Dreamers would benefit from eating more meat. A high-protein diet raises histamine, so the exception here would be for Stoic Dreamers who have histamine that is already too high and should moderate their protein intake. Star Dreamers, on the other hand, with their low histamine are particularly like to benefit from a high-protein diet.

The challenge then is to keep the diet moderate in fat in order to maintain a healthy heart and control cancer risk. Schizophrenic symptoms have also been associated with diets high in fat and/or saturated (animal) fat. In some remote regions of the Pacific Islands, schizophrenia is almost unknown, though there are some areas with a much higher prevalence. It turns out that in areas where the condition was very rare, the people ate mainly vegetables and fruits. In areas where schizophrenia was more common, fattier, Westernized diets were the norm (though they still contained no milk).

A more formal study looked at fat intake in the national average diet in eight different countries for correlations with the average occurrences of schizophrenia in each country. Those cultures with higher total fat (and higher saturated fat intake in particular) also had the most incidences of schizophrenia. Choosing lowfat sources of protein, then, is particularly important for Dreamers.

Caffeine is another frequent problem for Dreamers, because it exacerbates the Dreamer's excesses. Caffeine can cause or worsen anxiety, and the anxiety can make a person self-medicate, which can lead to ever-deepening anxiety. A study of hospitalized schizophrenic patients revealed that those who used the most caffeine tended to have the most psychotic symptoms. We know from animal studies that caffeine increases serotonin, a depression-fighting move that may account for some of its appeal. But it also increases dopamine, adrenaline, and noradrenaline. Remember, noradrenaline and adrenaline are excitatory neurotransmitters, and though they are generally beneficial, too much can cause overstimulation, pushing a Dreamer into trouble.

Essential Foods	Danger Foods
Grilled meat	Fruits
Vegetables	Sugar
Dairy products	Refined simple carbohydrates
Beans	Caffeine
Nuts	
Legumes	

Case in Point

Carol had her first breakdown about seven years before I met her. In addition to various compulsions, extreme fatigue, and seasonal depressions (particularly around the winter holidays), she had been diagnosed with psychotic depression. When she was in trouble, she was convinced that her black moods were a kind of personal persecution and that she was being punished for some terrible thing she had done. Carol had also suffered from an episode of postpartum psychosis after her daughter was born. During her depression, she was irrationally guilt-ridden, believing that she was somehow doomed for having given birth to a child.

She had many varied physical complaints, including burning sensations in her arms and neck, almost daily headaches, and eczema. She worried that she couldn't handle her social-work cases properly because her mind would get so blank at times that she couldn't read or concentrate on anything at all.

By the time Carol came to my office, she had already started taking niacin (vitamin B3) and was beginning to feel better as it cleared up her mental thought disorder. She'd had a glucose tolerance test done three years after the postpartum episode and was diagnosed as hypoglycemic, though the doctor who had ordered the test hadn't made any corrective suggestions. The basic lab tests I did were otherwise unremarkable.

Carol started on the usual hypoglycemic diet and took pyridoxine (vitamin B6) and zinc, with magnesium, thiamine, and brewer's yeast (for all the B vitamins) to help her body use the large doses of B6. Her depression and fatigue lifted, and she started to dream, or to remember her dreams, for the first time in years.

As I reviewed Carol's diet to help her discover where she needed to make changes, I noticed that she ate wheat products several times a day. Food allergies, or sensitivities, can contribute to nega-

(continued)

Case in Point *(continued)*

tive mental and emotional symptoms. In one study, schizophrenic patients had more antibodies (a sign of allergic reaction) than did control patients in reaction to a wide variety of tested foods. Milk and wheat (or more specifically, gluten, a protein found in wheat, barley, rye, and buckwheat) are especially likely to be culprits, which is why Carol's fondness for wheat alarmed me.

A thorough mental health workup should include ruling out food sensitivities as the source of the problem. So I suggested that Carol try a simple self-test. Per my advice, she avoided wheat entirely for five days. On the sixth day, she took her pulse before she got out of bed (68 beats per minute) and again when she was ready to eat breakfast (70 beats per minute). Then, she ate a bowl of plain Cream of Wheat, prepared with water and a little salt—her "test breakfast." Twenty minutes later, she took her pulse again. An increase of more than 16 beats per minute is considered positive for a food allergy, and Carol's pulse was up to 92—an increase of 22 beats!

That was all it took to identify the true source of her problems. Carol gave up wheat and wheat products immediately. Not only did her mental symptoms go away, but her chronic skin problems, which included stubborn eczema, also cleared up. On the wheat-free diet, Carol eventually stopped needing the megadose supplements and switched to a simple, high-quality multivitamin just once a day.

Of course, eliminating wheat wasn't an easy task for Carol, especially since it was such a large part of her diet. It might seem to reveal a twisted sense of humor on the part of Mother Nature that we become allergic to what we're addicted to. The very thing we eat most can end up causing the most problems. I think of it as the body's way of alerting us that we're overdoing a good thing.

(continued)

Case in Point *(continued)*

The benefits of cleaning up her diet were crystal clear to Carol, and this kept her on course. Once she recognized wheat's negative effects on her body, she also realized that she tended to turn to wheat foods in particular when she was under stress. To cut down on stress, she eventually decided to leave her job to raise her child full-time, thereby bypassing what was for her a rending conflict between work and parenthood. With a large portion of her daily stress gone, she found that she didn't feel so compelled to overeat in general any more, or to overeat wheat in particular.

Like many people with food allergies, Carol found that she could tolerate the offending food when she was feeling good physically and psychologically—and, when she was feeling good, she kept what she ate under much better control anyway. But when she was upset and stressed, the problem would reassert itself or intensify. In the past, that mechanism had led to raging psychosis over what might have been a rather ordinary temporary upset to a chemically balanced person. But now the spiral was a positive one: She was upset less, so she ate less wheat, so she was upset less, so the wheat she did eat bothered her less, so she was upset less—and so on.

The Dreamer Diet

The following is an outline of how Dreamers should eat to bring out their best. Additional advice for the particular subtypes appears at the end. This plan is designed primarily to balance your brain chemistry, but I want to note that following it, in combination with reasonable physical activity, will also help you control your weight and stay healthy in general. For our purposes, it isn't necessary to count calories or precisely measure what you eat in any way. All you need to keep track of is the rough number of servings of food you get in a few different categories.

Information on specific food choices appears in the chart below. (Foods not mentioned, and not included in the text as what you should avoid, are basically neutral and fine to include. Just about all vegetables are good, for example, though the ones mentioned in the chart have particular benefits.) First, however, I want to give you the outline of your eating plan:

- 5–7 small meals a day
- 3–4 servings lean animal protein
- 3–5 servings legumes, nuts, and seeds (vegetable protein)
- 7–11 servings of vegetables
- 5–6 servings whole grains
- 1 serving of fruit (optional)

(Stoic Dreamers should follow a slightly different pattern, as described in the section on that subtype on page 267.)

FOOD	BEST CHOICES	GOOD CHOICES	AVOID
Animal protein (lean) (3–4 servings)	beef chicken fish dairy products eggs salmon	tuna clams crab pork	processed dairy and meats
Legumes, nuts, and seeds (3–5 servings)	soybeans soy products (soy burgers, tofu, etc.) lima beans sunflower seeds	garbanzo beans (chickpeas) lentils navy beans cashews peanuts walnuts	canned beans in sugar sauce
Vegetables (7–11 servings)	asparagus peas spinach	alfalfa sprouts avocados broccoli Brussels sprouts cabbage carrots	canned or frozen vegetables with added sugar, EDTA, or preservatives

FOOD	BEST CHOICES	GOOD CHOICES	AVOID
		cauliflower collards green vegetables kale lettuce mustard greens parsley peppers potatoes tomatoes	
Fruit (1 serving, optional)	lemons limes grapefruit bananas oranges	apricots berries cherries guava grapes kiwi mangoes melons papaya pineapple raisins strawberries	overripe fruit (encourages candidiasis)
Whole Grains (5–6 servings)	wheat bran brown rice	shredded wheat cereal whole wheat rice polish wheat germ	white flour white rice
Sweeteners		honey maple syrup	white sugar chocolate refined sweeteners
Beverages	milk	water tomato juice	caffeinated drinks (including coffee, tea, sodas, and diet sodas)
Condiments and Seasonings	brewer's yeast		baker's yeast

Borderline Dreamers should follow the diet in the previous table.

When depressed, Star Dreamers will benefit from serotonin-promoting foods, including avocados, eggplant, tomatoes, and walnuts. If you are choosing to eat a serving of fruit, then bananas, pineapple, and plums are your best choices. These same foods should be avoided during an upswing.

Warrior Dreamers should add a few things to their "Best Choices" list (some of these have simply been upgraded from the general "Good Choices" list):

Animal protein
poultry
red meat
turkey (especially dark meat)
herring
oysters

Legumes, seeds, and nuts
black beans
almonds
pumpkin seeds and other squash seeds
pecans

Vegetables
kale
carrots
mushrooms
onions

Whole Grains
wheat germ
oatmeal

Finally, Stoic Dreamers have so many additions to make to the basic diet that I'm going to provide a whole new chart that incorporates the information in the chart above with the specifics appropriate for a Stoic Dreamer. Note also a few changes in the number of servings in the different categories.

FOOD	BEST CHOICES	GOOD CHOICES	AVOID

Animal protein (lean) (4–5 servings)	chicken
	turkey
	skim milk
	yogurt
	buttermilk
	cottage cheese
	cheddar cheese
	eggs
	salmon
	beef
	lamb
	halibut
	organ meats
		canned salmon
		  (with bones)
		canned sardines
		  (with bones)
		milk and dairy
		  products
		poultry
		herring
		oysters
		fish
		tuna
		pork
			shellfish
			sweetened
			  evaporated milk

Legumes, nuts, and seeds (2–4 servings)	almonds
	lima beans
	peanuts
	soybeans
	soy products (soy
	  burgers, tofu, etc.,
	  particularly tofu
	  made with cal-
	  cium (read labels)
	sunflower seeds
	walnuts
		garbanzo beans
		  (chickpeas)
		lentils
		navy beans
		cashews
		pumpkin seeds
		sesame seeds
		pecans
		black beans
		pinto beans
		pistachios
		kidney beans	

Vegetables (8–12 servings)	avocados broccoli eggplant peas spinach tomatoes potatoes	asparagus alfalfa sprouts Brussels sprouts cabbage carrots cauliflower collards green vegetables kale lettuce mustard greens onions parsley peppers tomatoes turnip greens	

FOOD	BEST CHOICES	GOOD CHOICES	AVOID
Fruit (1 serving, optional)	lemons limes grapefruit bananas pineapple plums	apples apricots berries cherries guava oranges kiwi mangoes melons papaya strawberries	dried fruit
Whole Grains (4–5 servings)	brown rice oatmeal corn or other whole grain tortillas	whole grain cereal whole grain bread	
Sweeteners		honey maple syrup (modest amounts) chocolate (only naturally sweetened, with honey or maple syrup)	white sugar refined sweeteners
Beverages			caffeinated drinks (including coffee, tea, sodas, and diet sodas)
Condiments and Seasonings	brewer's yeast iodized salt		cocoa

Brain Chemistry Markers

Several brain chemistry markers are useful in this type, as you'll see below, but there is no typical biochemical profile of the Dreamer in trouble. The only common ground is that, whatever the results, they are usually extreme. But one Dreamer may be extremely high on a particular marker, while the next Dreamer may be extremely low. If you are a Dreamer in trouble, you'll need to work closely with a doctor.

That should give you insight into why Dreamers in trouble are so difficult to fathom, but in case you need more convincing, there are at least four subtypes of Dreamers in trouble, and at least five important brain chemistry markers which, in various combinations, delineate each of them. Furthermore, Dreamers may show high or low scores in many of those markers. In fact, what is more important than the direction of the change from normal is the size of the change: Dreamers tend to have extreme scores, whatever the direction. To top it all off, some Dreamers in trouble have normal scores across the board—leaving good old-fashioned informed intuition as the best bet for knowing how to bring their brain chemistries into balance.

In short, for Dreamers, diagnosis is the hard part. Once it is done, treatment is just a matter of fact, matching solutions to symptoms and signs. Understanding yourself as a Dreamer, and knowing your subtype, leads you directly to the changes you need to make to avoid the pitfalls of your profile in trouble.

The main brain chemistry markers for all Dreamers are histamine, serotonin, blood sugar, copper, zinc, and thyroid hormone, so you should talk to your doctor about getting tested for your levels of these markers. (See Chapter 4: The Guardian for the components of a complete workup.) Because of the way Dreamers vary from one extreme to the other, we'll look at each of these as they pertain to particular Dreamer subtypes.

First, we'll look at the six vitamin deficiencies that have been linked to Dreamer-in-trouble behavior. As such, niacin, vitamin C, thiamine (vitamin B1), pyridoxine (vitamin B6), folic acid, and cobalamin (vitamin B12) are brain chemistry markers and are worth testing for. They are most useful in determining which therapies are most promising for bringing any given individual Dreamer into nutritional balance. Let's consider them, taking the more common first.

Normal Levels for Brain Chemistry Markers

Histamine	18–164 ng/ml
Serotonin	55–260 ng/ml (nanograms per milliliter)
Copper	68–143 mcg/dl
Zinc	60–130 mcg/dl
Thyroid hormone (thyroxine)	4.5–12.5 mcg/dl

NIACIN (VITAMIN B3)

Niacin deficiency is, in my experience, the most common vitamin-deficiency cause of imbalanced brain chemistry in Dreamers. Actually measuring the vitamin level may be deceptive, however, since, except in the severest deficiencies, the blood vitamin level will appear normal. I rely on psychological and physical signs and symptoms instead.

The first noticeable symptoms of niacin deficiency are entirely psychological. Victims may feel fearful, apprehensive, suspicious, and unable to concentrate. They worry excessively, with a gloomy, downcast, angry, and depressed outlook. They may experience headaches, insomnia, weakness, and burning sensations all over the body. Niacin-deficient people just fall apart under stress or go to extremes to avoid even the normal stresses of life. Niacin deficiency may dull the moral senses, causing promiscuity, lying, or petty thievery.

In mild deficiency, the tip of the tongue is usually reddened from engorgement with blood, and the taste buds on the tongue's surface are enlarged, giving a stippled appearance, the characteristic "strawberry tip." Farther back, the tongue is coated white with bacterial growth and debris, often giving off a foul mouth odor. As the deficiency becomes chronic, deep midline cracks and crevices appear. Later, the tongue becomes red and swollen all over, accompanied by dental indentations of the margins, lending it a scalloped appearance. Finally, the enlarged taste buds atrophy, and the tongue's surface develops a glossy, bald appearance. The mouth becomes sore and the gums swollen and painful. In mild niacin deficiency, digestive disturbances are also present. There is little or no secretion of hydrochloric stomach acid, absorption of nutrients is impaired, and the person has excessive gas and poorly formed, foul-smelling stools. In severe niacin shortage, symmetrical skin rashes develop on exposed areas, such as a butterfly-shaped rash on the cheeks.

VITAMIN C

Mental symptoms of vitamin C deficiency include fatigue, listlessness, lassitude, confusion, and depression. The face can have a haggard, frowning, "pained" expression and a careworn, knitted brow. Physical signs of scurvy (severe vitamin C deficiency) include a sallow or muddy complexion, breathlessness, disinclination for exercise, loss of appetite, anemia, desire for sleep, fleeting pains in the joints and limbs (especially legs,) bruising, sore gums that bleed readily, reddish spots, and hemorrhages on the skin.

THIAMINE (VITAMIN B1)

Mental symptoms of thiamine shortage include apathy, confusion, emotional instability, depression, a feeling of impending doom, fatigue, insomnia, and headaches. Physical signs include indigestion, diarrhea or constipation, poor appetite, weight loss, numbness or burning in the hands or feet, inability to tolerate pain, sensitivity to noises, low blood pressure, anemia, low metabolism, shortness of breath, heart palpitations, and an enlarged heart on X rays.

PYRIDOXINE (VITAMIN B6)

Pyridoxine deficiency can cause nervous symptoms and "emotionally upset" depression. People without enough vitamin B6 are often reclusive and shy but are free from delusions and hallucinations. Mild anemia is usually present and can be corrected with B6 supplements. Low blood sugar is especially common, causing headaches, dizziness, irritability, inability to concentrate, and extreme weakness. Excessive body weight, much of which is retained water, is shed quickly by pyridoxine's diuretic action.

A B6 deficiency may cause dandruff and oily scales on the scalp, eyebrows, around the nose, and behind the ears. Sufferers may experience numbness and cramping in the arms and legs. Their hands may be dry, cracked, and ache painfully, while their mouth and tongue are also cracked and sore. Nausea, especially in the morning, insomnia, and irregular periods in women are other prominent symptoms. Vitamin B6 increases mental imaging, so people who never or rarely dream or those who don't remember their dreams should suspect a B6 deficiency.

FOLIC ACID

Early in my practice, folic acid deficiency was the most common one I personally documented and was present in nearly 20 percent of my patients. Lately, given all the publicity about folate's ability to prevent birth defects, I find shortages more rarely. Mental symptoms of folic acid deficiency include poor memory, apathy, withdrawal, irritability, and slowing of the intellectual processes. Deficiency is particularly likely in the elderly (one study of older people found a shortage in 67 percent of participants) and should be suspected in any case of senility. Seizure medication such as Dilantin and myselin destroys folic acid, which means epileptics must be particularly careful to get sufficient amounts. Cracks and scaling on the lips and at the corners of the mouth can indicate folate shortage, as well as a big blood cell (macrocytic) or "pernicious" anemia. Like niacin and vitamin B12 deficiencies, lack of folic acid creates a vicious cycle by preventing digestive acid production and destroying the lining of the small intestine, creating malabsorption.

COBALAMIN (VITAMIN B12)

As with folic acid, vitamin B12 shortage causes a big blood cell anemia, pernicious anemia, which is ultimately fatal if uncorrected. A chronic untreated B12 deficiency results in neurologic degeneration, with numbness, tingling, unsteady gait, and loss of reflexes, among other things. Three to five years before the anemia or neurological changes, almost any type of mental symptom may appear, including apathy, mood swings, poor memory, disturbances in concentration and learning, hearing "voices," confusion, paranoia and psychosis, and especially senile psychosis. B12 deficiency was found in 58 percent of 138 such cases of psychosis and organic brain syndrome, and the late great mental health expert Carl C. Pfeiffer said that schizophrenia-like symptoms first appearing in middle or old age are usually due to B12 deficiency. A lack of B12 makes the tongue smooth at the tip and sides, and a glossy, beefy red all the way back.

Natural Medicine Solutions

I recommend several daily supplements to keep Dreamers in peak condition. The vitamin and mineral supplements (with the exception of iodine and lithium) discussed here are meant for daily use. They will boost the effects of a proper diet but, on the other hand, cannot do their work fully if the diet is not balanced. The amino acids, accessory nutrients, iodine, and lithium are for use in rebalancing your biochemistry when you are in trouble and are not intended for daily use over the long term. Once you get your diet under control and are in the habit of using the daily vitamins and minerals, these interventions should be unnecessary. Where there is a range of doses, the lower doses are meant for prevention and maintenance, while the higher levels are therapeutic for when you are in trouble. As always, take only what you need.

Mainstream psychiatry has little to offer that helps Dreamers in trouble. In the best-case scenarios, powerful drugs control symptoms, though they are not without potentially debilitating side effects of their own. For Dreamers in trouble, more than any other type, the natural medicine solutions offered here may be the best solution.

For information on using natural treatments at the same time as prescriptions, see p. 102.

We'll begin with a nutrient beneficial for all Dreamers, then break up the other supplements into groups for each Dreamer subtype. No matter what your subtype, you should read through all the suggestions to see if any apply to your situation and your brain chemistry markers. All are summarized in the table below, though not every supplement is appropriate for every subtype or every marker level.

DAILY SUPPLEMENTS	INTERVENTIONS	
	Amino Acids	Minerals
Vitamin C	Tryptophan	Lithium
B complex	5-HTP	
Niacin (vitamin B3)	Methionine	
Thiamine (vitamin B1)	Tyrosine	
Folic acid		
Pyridoxine (vitamin B6)		
Cobalamin (vitamin B12)		
Zinc		
Calcium		
Magnesium		
Manganese		

DAILY SUPPLEMENTS

For the Dreamer, taking these supplements regularly can keep your brain chemistry humming along, even in the face of stress or challenges. They can also be helpful, sometimes in higher doses, for Dreamers in trouble. What we know about them from a scientific viewpoint comes from studies of people out of balance, however.

Folic Acid

Folic acid is often deficient, or borderline deficient, in Dreamers in trouble, particularly where histamine is low. Deficiency in folic acid can cause schizophrenic symptoms, dementia, and psychosis, as well as depression.

Taking folic acid supplements can help raise low histamine levels. Folic

---

Folic Acid

RDA: 200 mcg daily. However, even conservative mainstream recommendations now call for at least 400 mcg a day, particularly for women of childbearing age, as sufficient folic acid is necessary for the prevention of neural tube birth defects.

Recommended Dose (general): 800 mcg–2 mg

Recommended Dose (in trouble): 1–20 mg daily with B12 and zinc

Maximum safe level: Unknown. Levels of 40 mg a day have been used without toxicity.

Contraindications: Don't take if you have gout or epilepsy. Consult with your doctor if you are taking medications for epilepsy.

---

acid is also a useful adjunct to other therapies. In one study, nearly all of the schizophrenic patients who were low in folic acid and took supplements along with standard treatment recovered, compared to just under 70 percent of those on standard treatment alone. Those who took the folic acid also improved more rapidly.

If you take folic acid supplements, you should always take cobalamin (vitamin B12) as well. Taking only folic acid could theoretically mask a deficiency in the B12, and B12 deficiency in particular can be devastating.

Niacin (vitamin B3)

Like anyone else, depressed Dreamers will benefit from niacin because of its ability to raise blood serotonin (see page 71 in Chapter 3: The Stoic). But some studies indicate that schizophrenic symptoms themselves may also be relieved by this B vitamin in pharmacologic doses. Niacin can help organize disordered thinking, including calming hallucinations and delusions.

The combination of niacin with standard treatments (whether drugs, therapy, or electroshock) showed the most dramatic effects in schizo-

Niacin

RDA (men): 18 mg

    (women): 13 mg

Recommended Dose (general): for men: 100 mg daily

                                          for women: 60 mg daily

Recommended Dose (in trouble): 500–3,000 mg daily

Maximum safe level: Any dose that does not cause diarrhea, vomiting, or bowel upset is safe.

Contraindications: Do not take niacin if you are taking high blood pressure medication, as it could make your pressure go too low. Don't take if you have ulcers, gout, or active liver disease or a liver disorder. Since niacin raises blood sugar, diabetics should consult with their doctors about managing their insulin dose before taking niacin.

---

phrenic patients compared to placebo. With niacin, patients were symptom-free more often and for longer periods, and required fewer hospitalizations as a group. People with close relationships and a solid work history seemed to improve most with niacin, according to one analysis of a group of many studies (though, that is surely a good recipe for healing no matter what sort of trouble you are in or what else you do about it).

Studies have shown that people with schizophrenic symptoms may not get as much niacin in their diets as healthy people, so niacin may work simply by correcting a deficiency. Niacin therapy increases mental serenity in all types of brain problems.

Stars and Dreamers in trouble sometimes have a similar pattern of overexcitement, showing low histamine and/or high serotonin. But they should use niacin in different ways. While Stars need moderate amounts and don't benefit by taking even more, a Dreamer in trouble should take larger doses.

Manganese

Manganese deficiency can cause schizophrenic symptoms, and studies have shown that schizophrenic patients have lower levels of the mineral, on average, compared to control groups.

Manganese supplements also help reduce copper overload. Nearly 60 percent of psychotic patients in one study improved after ten weeks on manganese (though schizophrenics without psychosis didn't show the same improvement). One study showed taking manganese tripled copper excretion in people with high copper (and low histamine). Results obtained by the same researchers using a combination of manganese and zinc were even better.

With my patients, I use 6–12 drops a day of a liquid solution I have specially prepared that is 10 percent zinc sulfate and .5 percent manganese chloride. That's good for those who don't have enough zinc or those who simply have too much copper. You can buy separate supplements of each, or look for combination capsules.

Manganese may increase blood pressure, especially in people older than forty, or cause headaches. Manganese toxicity can mimic manganese-deficiency symptoms.

Manganese

Recommended Dose (general): 2–5 mg daily

Recommended Dose (in trouble): 5–50 mg daily

Maximum safe level: Unknown

Contraindications: Unknown

Pyridoxine (Vitamin B6)

Not every Dreamer in trouble will respond to vitamin B6 supplements, but for those who do, it can be a beneficial treatment. Birth control pills can cause a B6 deficiency, so women using oral contraceptives who are experiencing psychiatric symptoms should be sure to take a B6 supplement. Studies show improvement in most cases with just 50 mg a day.

Vitamin B6

RDA (men): 2 mg

   (women): 1–6 mg

Recommended Dose (general): 10–50 mg daily

Recommended Dose (in trouble): 100–1,000 mg daily under physician supervision

Contraindications: If you're taking L-dopa (as for Parkinson's), check with a doctor before using vitamin B6 supplements.

Vitamin B6 and zinc seem to work well in tandem. Dreamers in trouble with low levels of these nutrients also generally have fair complexions, stretch marks, white spots on their fingernails, and low blood sugar.

Those deficient in B6 also tend not to remember their dreams. For these people, B6 improves mental imagery while sleeping, as well the memory of it. As part of your total daily dose, start with 50 mg at bedtime, and increase the dose after a few nights until you get dream recall (which in some people takes up to about 400 mg). B6 works best in combination with zinc (80 mg zinc sulfate a day for two months, then 30 mg a day for maintenance) and magnesium (400 mg a day).

Studies of patients with schizophrenic symptoms in general showed good results from combining B6 and niacin (vitamin B3), including some patients who required lower doses of tranquilizers. Patients taking the two in combination did better than those on either alone.

Start at 100 mg daily, and increase until you see some improvement. Check for dreaming and dream recall for indication you are getting enough. Don't exceed 500 mg daily, unless you are being treated by a knowledgeable physician.

Zinc

Zinc helps Dreamers in trouble by decreasing copper overload, rebalancing the copper to zinc ratio closer to the ideal 1:1, and alleviating symptoms. In

> ## Zinc
>
> **RDA:** 15 mg
>
> **Recommended Dose (general):** 30 mg daily
>
> **Recommended Dose (in trouble):** 80–160 mg for a few weeks at a time, in manic crisis.
>
> **Maximum safe level:** Unknown; one boy who consumed 12,000 mg (12 grams) zinc overslept for four days, fell asleep frequently through the day, wrote in illegible scrawl, staggered when he walked. Completely recovered by sixth day, no permanent harm.
>
> **Contraindications:** Unknown

one study, patients who excreted the most copper in their urine (while taking a mineral supplement and following a diet low in copper) showed the most improvement.

Some people experience nausea or excessive sweating with zinc, while for others it can make depression or hallucinations worse. Epileptics should consult with their doctors before using zinc.

Vitamin C

Dreamers in trouble need from 1–30 g (30,000 mg) daily. You can continue to raise the dose until maximum improvement occurs. Lower or discontinue the dosage if there is diarrhea or gastrointestinal upset.

> ## Vitamin C
>
> **RDA:** 45 mg
>
> **Recommended Dose (general):** 1,000–3,000 mg daily
>
> **Recommended Dose (in trouble):** 1,000–30,000 mg, use mineral ascorbate to avoid distention
>
> **Maximum safe level:** Unknown

STOIC DREAMERS

INTERVENTION

Tryptophan

Studies have shown that tryptophan improves the performance of lithium in treating schizophrenia. Other work shows that it does help stabilize mood in people with schizophrenic symptoms, though it probably does not address the disorder itself. Some studies indicate tryptophan is most effective in hostile, aggressive patients—most likely because it is calming.

The other supplements and interventions appropriate for Stoic Dreamers are the same as those covered in Chapter 3: The Stoic, and you should refer to that chapter for details.

Natural Medicine Solutions for Stoic Dreamers

To lower histamine:
Calcium: 500 mg twice a day *and*
Methionine: 500 mg twice a day

To raise serotonin:
Niacin: 1–6 g a day
5-Hydroxy Tryptophan (5-HTP): 200–300 mg at bedtime *or*
tryptophan: 1–3 g a day

To stabilize blood sugar:
Niacin: 100 mg three times a day
Zinc: 30–60 mg daily
Balanced B Complex: containing 50–100 mg of each B vitamin

To help normalize thyroid function:
Tyrosine: 1,500 mg daily
Balanced B Complex: 1–2, twice a day
Thiamine: 500–1,000 mg daily
Colloidal Iodine: 150 mcg daily
Magnesium: 400 mg daily

Tryptophan

Recommended Dose (in trouble): 500–9,000 mg a day.

Recommended Dose (for insomnia): 500–1,500 mg

Maximum safe level: Unknown. Don't exceed 3 grams a day unless you are under a doctor's close supervision. Theoretically, if L-tryptophan raises serotonin too high, *serotonin syndrome* can result, characterized by confusion, fever, shivering, sweating, diarrhea, muscle spasms, and, very rarely, death.

Contraindications: Don't drive or operate heavy machinery. Don't take with an antidepressant drug without discussing it with your doctor first.

STAR DREAMERS

INTERVENTIONS

Cobalamin (Vitamin B12)

Vitamin B12 also helps raise histamine levels. In cases where schizophrenia arises because of B12 deficiency, supplemental B12 can sometimes even be a cure.

Deficiency of vitamin B12 can cause schizophrenic symptoms, as well as confusion, memory loss, hallucinations, delusions, and paranoia.

B12 deficiency can cause mental symptoms as much as three to five years before the appearance of the grossly enlarged red blood cells that are the hallmark of the condition. That's one reason the road to a proper diagnosis is often a tortuous one. B12 deficiency is also often heralded by a host of aches and pains that accumulate gradually and can't be attributed to any particular cause—until the diagnosis is made.

Though B12 is present in all animal foods, especially liver, you can't generally eat your way to therapeutic doses because the deficiency is usually linked to an inability to absorb the vitamin in the gut. So B12 taken orally

Case in Point

Catherine was a top performer at her stressful, high-pressure academic job, managing a number of people and projects. But every now and then, when the voices she heard became more insistent and the delusions more bizarre, she'd make arrangements to check into a psychiatric hospital—carefully choosing one far enough from her home and workplace that she'd never run into anyone she knew. Catherine was unusually rational, organized, communicative, and verbal for a Dreamer in trouble, and she generally related to other people well. Once the stress got to be too much, though, she'd recognize when she was about to break down, and "check out" (by checking in) before it ever became too bad. For her, the hospital was a sanctuary, a respite from the stress of her work and a place of rest. She also got three square meals a day there, even if it was hospital food. At least there were no sugary sweets and no alcohol—her usual downfalls. She could also get higher doses of her medications in the hospital and have them readjusted for her outside life. In about a week, she would recover her grip on reality, and then she'd reenter the fray.

She'd managed this way for about seven years before I met her. She didn't feel she could go on in that way any longer. She came to me seeking an alternative.

Catherine's adrenaline level was very high, which correlated with the tremendous anxiety she was feeling. She had been taking lithium for years, so I was concerned about the depressed thyroid function that lithium can cause. I also suspected a deficiency of folic acid because the tranquilizer her original doctor had prescribed can cause them and because these deficiencies are frequently associated with schizophrenic symptoms.

The first thing I did was have her start on supplements of those

(continued)

vitamins. Though she said she felt better, she still got delusional and psychotic on occasion. So I added a regimen of high doses of niacin (she worked up from 3 to 8 g a day), which can be helpful in ordering thoughts and maintaining a sense of reality. I also added vitamin C, which discharges excessive adrenaline. With those, her constant fear (especially the fear that people could read her mind) dissipated. In heavy enough doses, vitamin C is an excellent natural tranquilizer, even for acute states. Catherine took 30 g a day.

Catherine also learned about the importance of an excellent diet, and whole, natural, unrefined foods. She never was a strict adherent, but still she made a lot of positive changes. And it was enough. On the high doses of niacin and vitamin C, she felt entirely well. As part of her own cure for herself, she left her high-powered job and now works low-key, part-time jobs. She eventually (and gradually) got off the drugs she'd taken for so long and has never needed hospitalization again.

Now the most positive aspects of her Dreamer profile have emerged, no longer eclipsed by the negative pull of the Dreamer in trouble. Her vision is to make the world understand what it is like to be schizophrenic. By fighting the stigma commonly attached to the Dreamer in trouble, she hopes to open the door for everyone to reach their own positive potential. The articles she's published are a legacy she's immensely proud of.

(in food or pills) isn't really available to the body anyway. B12 usually must be given by intramuscular injection with a doctor's prescription. The usual series is one 1,000 mcg/1 ml injection two to three times a week for two or three months. (To make this process more convenient, you can learn to give yourself the shot with a tiny needle.) When B12 deficiency is first detected, I usually recommend repeating the series of shots after a three-month break. Alternating three-month blocks with and without injections for one

> **Vitamin B12**
>
> RDA: 6 mcg daily (taken orally)
>
> Recommended Dose (general): 1,000 mcg daily (taken orally or sublingually)
>
> Recommended Dose (in trouble): 1,000 mcg by injection every 2–3 days for 2–3 months
>
> Maximum safe level: Unknown
>
> Contraindications: None

year is usually in order. For maintenance, one series every two years is usually sufficient. The body stores vitamin B12 for years, but it takes a while to rebuild your stores once they've dropped very low.

Fortunately most people see improvement in their mental symptoms early on in this process. Just as they are the first symptoms to appear, they are the first symptoms to abate with treatment. Improvement in physical symptoms often takes longer, and improvement in the size and shape of the blood cells still longer.

Malabsorption of vitamin B12 is genetically linked and is more common in those of Northern European backgrounds, especially those who are fair-haired and light-skinned. Heavy drinking can also destroy the body's ability to absorb vitamin B12. In fact, I've had patients who simply drank themselves into deficiency.

Most times when schizophrenic symptoms are due to deficiency in vitamin B12, other blood chemistry markers we've discussed are normal. But there are some people with other imbalances in addition to B12 shortage.

Lithium

Lithium is helpful to some, but not all, people with schizophrenia. Since lithium lowers serotonin, it is most likely to be useful in Star Dreamers in trouble who have excess serotonin.

Lithium aspartate

Recommended Dose (in trouble): 5 mg 1–8 times daily

Maximum safe level: Don't take more than 4 doses daily unless you are under a doctor's care.

Contraindications: Kidney or cardiovascular disease, dehydration, salt depletion

---

Case in Point

My secretary came to tell me I had better see a new patient, though his appointment wasn't for an hour yet. I found Paul lying in the front yard of my office, beating the ground with his fists, crying and moaning. When I coaxed him inside, I was not surprised to learn he had been hospitalized several times since falling ill three years before. He was miserable, he told me (though I might have guessed that) and depressed. He hallucinated sometimes, hearing voices in his head. His business was failing, he couldn't seem to form any new relationships, and he had nearly destroyed the ones he had.

In technical terms, he was in sorry shape. Though Paul wasn't taking any medication, most patients with problems similar to his are prescribed tranquilizers some time before they find their way to my office. I remember Paul so well because his was one of the fastest and most complete reversals of schizophrenic symptoms I have ever witnessed.

I gave him the full battery of tests, but almost everything came back normal. Everything, that is, except his routine blood test, which revealed serious anemia, with greatly enlarged red blood

(continued)

Case in Point *(continued)*

cells. Further testing pointed to malabsorption syndrome regarding vitamin B12, or borderline pernicious anemia.

Paul took a series of vitamin B12 shots to undo the deficiency, and his fearsome nature quickly dissolved. He was no longer psychotic. Now, able to converse rationally, Paul emerged as highly intelligent and filled with altruistic aims maintained from his younger days as a "hippie." To calm the voices that he heard when he was really out of control, he also took niacin, which can make thinking processes clearer and make the senses work better in general. To balance all the B12 he was taking, he took a good B-complex supplement (getting folic acid is especially important, as B12 works together with folic acid). Within six months, Paul's brain chemistry was stabilized. In similar cases, I might have prescribed a dose of GABA in times of overexcitement, but Paul's condition reversed so completely that he didn't even need that.

By then, he'd long escaped the zombie-self I first met there on my lawn. He was still an authentic Dreamer, with some "far out" Dreamer views—he was an idealist through and through, with radical political views. But as his moods stabilized, his business turned around, and his innate ability to be charming resurfaced. His social life in general revived, and he began dating again, apparently with much success. He was never hospitalized again for psychiatric causes.

Vitamin B12 deficiency can be much more stubborn to treat, and in many cases it takes the body much longer to recover than it did in Paul's case. And that's only once the problem has been identified. Pernicious anemia isn't always quickly or easily identified, as you might have guessed from the fact that it was never spotted in Paul's previous hospitalizations. Paul's case demonstrates, in part, the enormous benefit of catching and treating B12 deficiency as soon as possible.

Natural Medicine Solutions for Star Dreamers

To raise histamine:

Folic acid: 1 mg twice daily

Cobalamin (Vitamin B12): 1,000 mcg/ml intramuscular injection two to three times a week for two to three months. Though injections are preferred, oral or sublingual B12 also raises blood histamine.

Niacin: 3–6 g daily

To lower serotonin:

Lithium aspartate: 5 mg 1–12 times daily (don't use more than five times a day unless you are working with a health care practitioner)

WARRIOR DREAMERS

Natural Medicine Solutions for Warrior Dreamers

To balance high copper/raise zinc:

Zinc sulfate: 30 mg a day. Practitioners may prescribe up to 150 mg daily, but zinc can cause copper-deficient anemia at those levels, so megadoses should be taken only under medical supervision.

Manganese: 10 mg daily, or 30–60 daily only under the supervision of a health care practitioner, to treat tardive dyskinesia (a central nervous system disorder) side effect.

BORDERLINE DREAMERS

Natural Medicine Solutions for Borderline Dreamers

Vitamin C: 1–30 g

Pyridoxine (Vitamin B6): 100–500 mg

Mind/Body and Lifestyle Changes

Like all types, Dreamers will benefit from developing the best characteristics of other types, especially those next to and opposite from them on the pie chart (see p. 28) along with their own Dreamer strengths. That's the formula for ensuring *sweet* dreams.

I do talk therapy with almost all of the Dreamers I see, and our discussions tend to be particularly intense and intimate. Even after correcting their brain chemistry, they are still likely to benefit from psychotherapy. In this section, I'll describe the things that have helped me in my practice with Dreamers, so you can look for a therapist who works in similar ways. It can be tricky to find the therapist who is just the right match for you, but this can at least help make your search a little more efficient.

For Dreamers in trouble, a cure usually requires not only diet and nutrition (often all that is required for many other types) but lifestyle changes as well. The choices Dreamers make about what to do, how to behave, and who and what to surround themselves with are crucial, and Dreamers may need help focusing on the nuts-and-bolts practicalities of these matters, as well as the emotional and psychological aspects. Whether, why, and how to enter college, join a church, move, or change jobs can stymie a Dreamer, and at the same time are integral to creating a complete and supportive life. Here, again, the results are cyclical: Staying out of bad situations allows people to be kind to themselves, including eating healthfully, which helps them stay out of bad situations. And so on.

Stoic Dreamers do best in individual therapy, while Star Dreamers can thrive in group therapy. Borderline Dreamers are the exception here. I don't see them very often because they generally aren't looking for help. Their problems aren't serious enough to force them into it. When they do come to me, good nutrition is usually enough to rebalance them.

Supportive therapy is the most appropriate for Dreamers, because it focuses on material problems. Dreamers in trouble tend to be caught up with spiritual concerns and may need someone to remind them to simply eat, sleep, and groom themselves. The situation isn't always that severe, of course, but the needs are always practical. For Dreamers in trouble, a therapist is often also a dispenser of financial, organizational, social, and even housekeeping advice. Dreamers need to control the amount of stimuli in their lives, until there are no more external stresses than are manageable.

For Dreamers, that threshold is often low. And they might need help seeing *how* to do it. Most should start by knowing Dreamers do best in serene environments, working by themselves in low-pressure jobs. I've seen more Dreamers pushed into trouble by work that didn't suit them than I can count.

For Dreamers, a therapist should also function as a friend would. When they are deeply enmeshed in their own inner world and problems, Dreamers are often friendless. They've been rejected too often or may not even know how to make a friend. They might be estranged from their families or just have put even the most well-meaning family members through the wringer already, so they have nothing left to give. So Dreamers in trouble need casual, everyday support and advice—the kind they get from their social networks when they are in balance—as well as psychological and psychiatric expertise.

As far as the latter category, it mostly consists of me letting the Dreamer across from me do the talking. Dreamers are very smart, as I've said, and often have already done a lot of thinking on whatever topic is on their minds. In fact, they've usually *over*-thought it, to the point where the simplest thing can take on a life of its own.

My job then is to do "reality testing." I listen to their stories very carefully, and then ask them to go over it again—very carefully. Then I'll ask for clarifications: What did she really say? What were the exact words she used? Could there be any other explanation? Did you really see X, or could it have been a hallucination, as it has been in the past? Remember last time you thought something like this had happened, and it turned out to have a perfectly ordinary explanation? Answering these types of questions makes the person focus on the facts and draw his own conclusions from there. Dreamers will learn the extent to which their own negative expectations create their negative state. When they finally *know* that, they have motivation to set neutral or realistically positive expectations.

Building social support *outside* of the counseling office is another important aspect of treatment. The many community support groups devoted to allowing individuals with the same condition to share their common ex-

Paranoia, The Destroyer

For Dreamers in trouble who experience paranoia (or for those who irrationally feel the cards are stacked against them), three simple steps can help keep those impulses in check:

1. Always give the other person the benefit of the doubt.
2. Don't jump to false conclusions based on your own negative expectations. Go over the events you are upset about slowly and carefully, trying hard to recall exactly what was really said or done.
3. See the best in things. Assume somebody up there likes you and is trying to help you. When things go wrong, instead of believing "they" are out to get you, try assuming everything is for the best. Look for the cloud's silver lining.

Sometimes, of course, bad things do happen. Just make sure you know what is *actually* happening first, before wasting your energy in response. And don't be blind to the good things going on.

periences and feelings are one way to do this. They are a safe place to practice new coping skills and take emotional risks in a controlled environment. The ultimate goal is to create the same level of comfort in the "outside" world as well.

For that reason, I spent a lot of time helping Esther (see page 242) learn to reach out to people. She was extremely shy (most Dreamers are; it is part and parcel of being so intensely inner-directed). Making friends, like any other new skill, takes practice. So I gave her a "homework" assignment: Every time she passed someone in the halls at school, she was to smile and say "hi." That was it.

Esther came back to the next session saying she had to force herself to do it and complained that people would respond by looking at her quizzically, as if they were trying to determine how they knew her. They didn't always return her smile or greeting—but some did. Esther agreed to keep on with this strategy. By the next time I saw her, she was not only getting a response in kind more often than not but also was finding that people had begun to come up to her to say hello, without her ever having to say anything. To her it seemed miraculous. Once she got it working for her, she found she enjoyed this more open and receptive stance. As time went on, some of these acquaintances turned into true friendships.

ANGER

For Dreamers in trouble, anger is usually never very far away. Like Warriors, they react with anger when they sense a threat to their security. It's a defense against anxiety.

In Dreamers anger usually develops as a slow burn. They won't even notice they've been insulted at first (sometimes it's because they haven't been!), but they'll brood over whatever it was later, sometimes obsessively. They can't deal with it directly—that would be much too confrontational for their natures—and so it festers. Nothing good can come of this. They are just building up a huge head of steam with absolutely no vent: a recipe for an explosion, which is obviously destructive. The issue just roils their insides, tormenting them, growing ever larger and ever more significant, problematic, and intractable. In some Dreamers, this escalates into fantastical proportions. Dreamers are really the explosive type, so there's no escape except burrowing further inside. Too much of that means seriously warped perceptions—or even a loss of touch with reality.

It would behoove Dreamers to learn to be more Warriorlike in how they handle anger, recognizing what makes them angry and responding to it directly and emphatically. (Warriors in trouble sometimes take this to unfortunate extremes, but unless you are a Warrior, you never have to worry about going too far in that profile since it is a stretch for you in the first place.)

As with all brain types, Dreamers benefit from drawing on some traits from other types (as in the example about handling anger, above). Without ever losing their unique Dreamer-ness, many Dreamers come into balance when they get in touch with the Lover in themselves—the part that relates to others. Positive traits of other types can cover your trouble spots and play

Mirror, Mirror on the Wall

Your face is your window on the world, but it is also the world's window into you. For anyone struggling with interpersonal relationships, this easy exercise can yield surprising (and helpful) results:

Study yourself in the mirror. How do you look to others?

I had one patient who gave me dirty looks all the time she was with me. The conversation we were having was a tough one, granted, but I didn't think she really had such negative feelings toward me. So I asked her if she knew she was doing it. She didn't even believe she *was* doing it until she looked for herself. The fact was, she looked scary. For those who didn't know her, that expression was all they'd have to go on. It was even off-putting for those who did know her, who assumed she was always upset and angry with them, even when they couldn't see what they had done to deserve such treatment.

My suggestion to her (not that she liked it at first) and to you, was to practice a calmer expression. That is, literally standing in front of the mirror, examining the image you project to others, and making adjustments. The corners of my patient's mouth were always turned down, so she practiced holding the slightest of smiles. As I told her, it takes fewer muscles to smile than to frown. She also learned to take the wrinkles out of her brow, relaxing her forehead until they went away.

Until you try it yourself, you might not believe the effort this takes—or the benefits it brings. Some schools of thought hold that if you "act as if," what you are enacting will come true for you. I'm not sure myself that looking happy is all that it takes to make you happy. But it sure is harder to feel happy when you *look* mopey or angry. And I'm positive about the difference you'll see in how others react to you when you face the world with a pleasant expression.

up your strengths, allowing you to be the best Dreamer you can be. Like anything else, it will take practice. To "stay in shape," try some of the following strategies:

Join up. Belonging to an association based on common interests is the most natural way to relate to others. So whether it is a church, dance class, gardening club, or the PTA, become a member of something and participate in its regular activities. Any group you join will help keep your social skills from getting rusty. If you like, you could even try something like Toastmasters International, which is an organization specifically aimed at helping people develop social skills.

Go out. Socialize with friends. Go somewhere you've never been. Try something new. Choose something that interests you by all means, but get out there and interact with the larger world. Go to an actual movie rather than renting yet another video. Eat at a restaurant. Accept an invitation to a party.

Spruce up. Do something to improve your appearance. Buy some new clothes. Get a facial, haircut, or a manicure.

Speak out. When you are socializing, be aggressive (for you). Initiate conversations. Give more than one-word answers, even to yes or no questions. Talk to someone new.

An analogy I heard from Marty McCarthy, codirector of Transitional Living Services in Sacramento, has always stayed with me: "Most people are like Timex watches," she said. "They take a licking and keep on ticking. Still, it's a cheap, common watch."

A Dreamer, on the other hand, is like a fine Swiss watch, she says. Much better than a Timex. But if you bang it around, it will break. It is a precise, delicate instrument. When it's working properly, it is a work of art as well as engineering.

The Lover

8

Ardent, open-hearted, outgoing, attractive, enthusiastic, sensitive, compassionate, and radiant with sexual energy (even if it is sometimes unconscious); that's the Lover in balance. Lovers know how to enjoy life, and they live it to the fullest. They have a good time and bring those around them along for the ride. Lovers know how to make others feel good. They throw themselves wholeheartedly into whatever they are doing. They are charming, smooth, and sociable, often flirtatious, and easy to be around. You want Lovers at your dinner party. You could speak to a Lover for two minutes at a massively crowded gathering, and they'll make you feel like you're the only person in the room worth talking to. Lovers also tend to get their way.

For Lovers, relationships are, paradoxically, their strength and their weakness. Relationships assume such primary importance that some Lovers feel as if they literally don't exist except within one. That, not surprisingly, can lead to incredible anxiety centered on relationships—finding them, getting them, keeping them. But a Lover in balance, pouring their psychic energy into a healthy relationship, is a force of nature. That's the power of love.

The Lover is a common profile among celebrities, because they can reach across even space and time to make what feels like a personal connection. Live and in person, a Lover's magnetism is still unmistakable. It doesn't necessarily make them pinups or movie stars, but they can be equally compelling in a variety of fields. They shine wherever interpersonal connection is primary.

Lovers have strong emotions, so they avoid the emotional suppression of the Stoic type. They let you know what they are thinking and feeling. As long as that works on the level of "being in touch with" themselves and their emotions, this is a healthy aspect of the Lover profile. But it is also an Achilles' heel, leaving Lovers vulnerable to mood swings, excessive emotionalism (whatever the mood), depression, and, most commonly, anxiety (more about that later). Women are almost twice as likely as men to have anxiety, but men are more likely to resort to alcohol and drugs to cover it up.

Many Lovers are troubled by frustrations in love—as with Marilyn's early marriage (see box on p. 289), multiple short-lived subsequent marriages, infidelity, and frigidity. Lovers in trouble are often seductive and promiscuous. Out-of-balance male Lovers tend to be womanizers; females tend to have a weakness for the "bad boy" type. Both are fickle, with a little devil inside them constantly prodding them to see if the grass is greener elsewhere, no matter how good the current relationship.

What all Lovers are looking for, however, is not so much sex as security. Lovers are highly dependent on others; their security comes from feeling they are attractive to and loved by others. Their sense of self-worth, even their sense of self, is conditional on how much they feel loved. They are hypersensitive to criticism, tending to emotionally overreact to even the slightest perception of negativity. Lovers are very social and socially active, but Lovers in trouble might suffer from social anxiety. Lovers feel safe and secure only when they know they are desired. And when they feel their security is threatened, they become anxious.

THOSE WHO FORGET THE PAST . . .

A lot of Lovers try to change history by repeating it, an approach that is doomed to fail. They experience one failure after another, but in a way that's what they're subconsciously after. If they had a good relationship, it would be like saying those that rejected them early in their lives were no good. And they are not ready for that. They'd rather consider *themselves* no good. They don't feel worthy of a good relationship and are unlikely to have one until they do. Lovers are usually humble and modest, but sometimes those traits just hide extremely low self-esteem.

Lovers, like Warriors, tend to be amoral and deceptive when they are in trouble: "All's fair in love and war." Their main concern is getting what they want or need. For Lovers, this typically means acting the way another person wants them to be in order to secure and maintain a relationship. The strain of crafting every action to fit someone else's desires and never revealing your true self dooms any relationship based on it. Yet Lovers in trouble may be so desperate for the relationship and its illusion of security that they persist in this destructive "strategy."

Lovers in trouble must also be wary of the opposite problem: They tend to be easily deceived and taken advantage of, and unduly influenced by others' opinions.

Many Lovers in trouble become what psychiatry calls "anxiety hysterics." They may experience many different physical symptoms (the most common include headaches, gastrointestinal upset, and backaches) for which no organic cause can be found. Though all the profiles have a constellation of physical symptoms that improve when the underlying brain chemistry is corrected, complaints of aches and pains are de rigueur for Lovers.

Symbolically, this is an extension of their deceptive abilities, only this time, it is the ability to lie to themselves. That's not to say physical ailments aren't a very real experience—95 percent of pain is subjective. Anxiety lowers the threshold of pain, so Lovers who experience anxiety also experience any pain in an exaggerated form (in contrast to Dreamers, who tend to minimize and underreport symptoms of pain). As emotionally expressive people, Lovers are also simply more likely to identify and acknowledge pain. Low blood sugar also lowers the pain threshold, and I'm sure at this point it will come as no surprise to you when you review the recommended diet for Lovers in this chapter that low blood sugar is often what puts Lovers in trouble.

Emotionally facile as they can be, one feeling Lovers can't handle is anger. They often deal with anger by getting anxious. Suppressing anger (since no one can entirely avoid it) leads to the kind of somatic anxiety that sometimes manifests in muscle tension, rapid heart palpitations, dry mouth, profuse sweating, nausea, nervousness, and feelings of fear—in combination, a panic attack. Phobias are also relatively common in Lovers in trouble. At the extreme end of this path lies hysterical paralysis, amnesias, and even altered states of consciousness leading to dissociative states.

Even well before things get to that point (which they *very* rarely do), Lovers in trouble often fear that they are "going crazy." Guardians do, too. But take heart: People with either profile almost never do become insane. (Ironically, Dreamers and Stars, who can both become psychotic when they are very sick, are not usually the ones fearing madness. On the contrary, they will even deny it when they are.) I suppose this is why I've heard my colleagues who don't specialize in psychiatry jokingly sum up what they learned in med school about psychiatry this way: If you think you might be crazy, you're not.

ANXIETY

When Lovers are out of balance, the most common mental symptom is anxiety. And among Americans, anxiety is a fairly common disorder. About 65 million people suffer from anxiety each year. Just over half of them have a mild to moderate affliction, while the rest suffer from a full-scale, disabling disorder. One in two people have anxiety for at least two weeks at some time in their lives. Anxiety is also often linked with depression. In a 1997 Gallup Poll, fully a quarter of American workers reported facing anxiety and chronic stress. Yet less than 25 percent of people with anxiety get the help they need.

Anxiety has many forms, including panic attacks, phobias (including specific phobias, social phobia, and agoraphobia), post-traumatic stress disorder, obsessive-compulsive disorder, hypochondria, and the catchall "generalized anxiety disorder," or GAD. Anxiety can include fearful feelings, worry, uncertainty, apprehension, and unexplainable dread. It can manifest physically in many ways, primarily with symptoms related to arousal of the central nervous system, including shaking, muscle tension, restlessness, fatigue, nonspecific aches and pains, nausea or other gastrointestinal distress, shortness of breath, rapid or irregular heartbeat, sweating or clamminess, dry mouth, insomnia, headaches, hot flashes or chills, lightheadedness, trouble swallowing, frequent urination, edginess, concentration problems, and irritability. Anxiety can exacerbate other conditions, including overeating, alcoholism, PMS, or irritable bowel syndrome. An initial episode of anxiety rarely occurs after age forty-five.

Physiological causes of anxiety are described below, but everyday stresses are also important contributors. In fact, part of the medical definition of "generalized anxiety disorder" is unrealistic or excessive worry about life

Panic Attacks

One common and particularly disturbing form of anxiety is the panic attack. The symptoms are similar to generalized anxiety, but are particularly intense, begin all of a sudden, and peak within ten minutes before subsiding. Paralyzing fear and dread are typical, and panic attacks usually involve difficulty breathing, rapid heartbeat, chest pains, and dizziness. The feelings are so extreme, people often confuse them with heart attack symptoms or believe they are about to die.

Panic attacks may arise unexpectedly, but some people experience them consistently in certain circumstances (boarding an airplane, taking a test, being in a large crowd). Identifying situational triggers is one way to begin to find a solution, such as avoidance of the situation. In the likely event that avoidance isn't always possible, more productive ways to handle those situations can be identified as well.

circumstances. Common sources include work-related difficulties, grief, marital woes, health concerns, financial crises, and social fears. Some anxiety is a normal part of life, but when symptoms become serious enough to interfere with daily life, it qualifies as an anxiety disorder. Under the official definition of the American Psychiatric Association, 7 percent of adults in the United States have an anxiety disorder.

Anxiety and depression share many of the same symptoms, including irritability, guilt, fatigue, change in eating habits, sleep problems, chronic aches and pains, and inability to concentrate.

About one-half of people with anxiety are also depressed, and about one-third of depressed patients are also anxious. Approximately 12 million Americans face the combination, and telling the difference isn't always simple. For example, excessive worry, a hallmark of anxiety, is one of the ten most common symptoms of depression. When your brain chemistry is out of balance, getting an accurate picture of which you have—either or both—can help you accurately tailor your approach to regaining biochemical balance in your brain.

Type	General Traits	Beneficial Aspects	Harmful Aspects	Vulnerabilities
Lovers	Outgoing Attractive Empathic Loving Sexual Flirtatious Warm Emotionally expressive Sensitive Seductive	Live life to the fullest. Can count Marilyn Monroe as one.	Manipulate others. Are dependent. Are insecure. Can't handle anger. Practice deception. Are easily deceived. Act promiscuously. Are fickle. Are hypersensitive. Overreact. Fear rejection. Have low self-esteem. Are amoral. Lie to themselves. Have hypochondria.	Lovers in trouble tend to get anxious and are prone to panic attacks.

Case in Point

Norma's mother had a "nervous breakdown" when Norma was just beginning grade school. Consequently, her mother spent the rest of her life in and out of mental institutions. Norma's father had walked out on her mother (on Christmas Eve!) when she'd told him that she was pregnant, so Norma never knew him—or even knew if he was alive or dead. Even before her mother's hospitalization, Norma lived with a foster family because her single mother, working at a low-paying job, couldn't afford to take care of her. Norma spent most of her childhood bounced around among many different foster homes. Her mother, though essentially incapacitated until after Norma became an adult, would not give up custody and allow Norma to be adopted, though several kind-hearted families had offered. She could neither care for her nor let her go.

In one foster home, when she was eight years old, Norma was sexually abused by an elderly boarder and got slapped for lying when she reported the incident. In another home, when Norma was nine, her foster mother remarried suddenly and, without warning, packed up Norma's belongings and dropped her off at an orphanage.

As a young teenager, Norma was molested again and gave birth to a baby she was forced to put up for adoption. Another foster father once barged into her bedroom at night and kissed her passionately. Though the sexual crime proceeded no further, the humiliation was complete.

By her early teenage years, Norma was already buxom, beautiful, and adept at accentuating those facts and using them to her advantage. She was conveniently married off at sixteen—just when her then-foster mother was moving across the country. Norma soon began to have affairs while her husband, a Navy man, was stationed overseas. She began working as a "model," which included

(continued)

Case in Point *(continued)*

posing nude, and even occasionally worked as a call girl. Her marriage broke up after four years. By the time she was nineteen, she had made two suicide attempts.

This was the pre-pill era, and Norma went through a series of twelve abortions over the years, some of them in less-than-safe environments; she was a woman without resources at a time when the procedure was largely illegal. Finally, she had her tubes tied, but later regretted that decision and underwent still more surgery in an attempt to reverse the procedure. It should come as no surprise that she was often unable to enjoy sexual relationships.

Digging into Norma's childhood, I wasn't greatly surprised to learn any of this, because I already knew the end of the story: two more short-lived marriages, paralyzing performance anxiety, torrid affairs, and, finally, a barbiturate overdose amid swirling rumors of foul play. She also had fabulous fame and riches as possibly the greatest sex symbol of all time, for Norma is better known to the world as Marilyn Monroe. Her public image is the epitome of the Lover profile, while her private life models the psychological underpinning of the type in trouble.

Marilyn never found a comfortable way to integrate these parts of herself, and though I only knew her as a larger-than-life figure on the screen, and not as a patient, I suspect out-of-balance brain chemistry could have been to blame. She had tragedy enough in her life, to be sure, but was also blessed with amazing personal power. I don't think it was just her legs or breasts or platinum blonde hair or provocative poses that made her a legend. Other stars before and since have had similar combinations, but no one else has retained such a grip on the public imagination. I wonder what extraordinary life she might have lived if she could have been

(continued)

Case in Point *(continued)*

simply the Lover, like her public image, rather than the Lover in trouble she couldn't seem to escape in real life.

Not all accounts of Marilyn Monroe's life agree on all the incidents of sexual abuse recounted above, but these are all stories Marilyn herself told at one time or another. Some other details about her sexual history, particularly the adoption offers, abortions, and lack of sexual interest are also not agreed on by all sources. The exact truth will probably never be known, but I've included these stories, even at the risk of passing along something unsubstantiated, because I think they make an important point about her life. The simplest view—that these stories are true—helps explain why Marilyn was always a Lover in trouble. Even if they are not all documentable—even if she was just spinning horrific fantasies—the messages the stories carry of the danger and humiliation of sex; the confusion of sex and love; and the constant threat of rejection, betrayal, and abandonment, all make the same point.

Dietary Guidelines

The high-protein, low-sugar, and small, frequent meals diet is good for all Lovers and is crucial for Lovers with hypoglycemia. As always, avoiding refined foods, and particularly white sugar and white flour, is important for getting all the nutrients you need. For Lovers, avoiding caffeine and other stimulants (including nicotine), as well as alcohol, is also important.

We commonly think of sugar as giving us "energy." We already know it stimulates us in the same way that nervousness and anxiety do. When we are otherwise in balance we might call it being "wired," "hyper," or "buzzed," but if we aren't perfectly poised to handle the spike in blood sugar, those same feelings can translate into anxiety. Diets high in white sugar have been linked to higher rates of anxiety, and sugar has been proven to be able to cause nervousness, headaches, and even panic attacks in people who are susceptible in those things. Eliminating refined sugar has been shown to reduce anxiety.

Sugar increases energy and improves mood—it can even relieve mild anxiety. It also directly stimulates neurons in the brain, because sugar provides ready and quick food for the brain. The catch—and it is a big one—is that the sugar is quickly used up, and when the blood sugar level drops, so does serotonin. The change is often steep, and you're left with feelings of fatigue, depression, and/or anxiety.

If you're using sugar—consciously or unconsciously—to relieve anxiety, you may be getting fast but very short-lived results. You're also making the original problem even worse every single time. A snack of complex carbohydrates from whole foods can help calm and relax you without putting you on that downward spiral. It may take a bit longer to feel the effects, but once they do appear, they should last a few hours rather than a few minutes. For general health, you want to make sure what you eat is low in fat. That doesn't include dairy fats like butter, cheese, and whole milk, which are beneficial in moderate amounts.

Danger Foods

Refined foods
White flour
Sugar, especially white
Caffeine and other stimulants
Nicotine
Alcohol

Despite all the problems in her life, Marilyn herself did do one important thing that probably saved her from feeling even worse: she exercised. To keep herself in shape, she was known to lift weights and run every morning. And this was at least thirty years before such activities became popular, par-

Calming Foods

Did you know that you can find benzodiazepines—which are used as tranquilizing drugs that commonly combat anxiety—in many common foods? You'd have to eat more than humanly possible at any given time to get the equivalent of one dose of Valium. But you might try emphasizing these foods in your diet to get some benefits.

Lentils
Soybeans
Rice
Corn
Potatoes
Cherries
Mushrooms

ticularly for women. She must have been born with a strong physical constitution, and she did her bit to maintain it, despite her apparent drug and alcohol abuse.

CAFFEINE

Along with sugar, Lovers must avoid all other stimulants, which only serve to initiate or exacerbate anxiety. For most people, that really means to steer clear of caffeine. Caffeine can cause severe anxiety or set off full-blown panic attacks. One study even created panic attacks in people who'd never had one before by dosing them with caffeine (albeit in extremely large quantities).

Caffeine works on the central nervous system, increasing activity of the neurotransmitters, so that it can improve mood. But that immediate effect disappears quickly, and within hours, anxiety, nervousness, and muscle tension replace any initial boost. The more dramatic the effect a substance has on you in the short run, the bigger the whiplash you're likely to experience in terms of getting the opposite effect over the long haul. Along with sugar, caffeine is the most obvious example of this effect.

Anxiety-prone people (like Lovers) are often more sensitive to caffeine than other people. Perhaps there's something genetic that makes a person more susceptible to stress and to caffeine or that magnifies reactions until they are out of proportion. In any case, in sensitive people, just five cups of coffee is probably enough to instigate an attack. (That's in official six-ounce cups, by the way, so that grande latte you're sipping probably gets you more than half-way there.)

The good news is that simply eliminating caffeine can eliminate the anxiety or stop the panic attacks. There's bad news, though: Caffeine withdrawal can cause anxiety, too. Keep in mind that withdrawal is a time-limited effect, and the long-term benefits will be more than worth it. But it might help to eliminate your caffeine intake gradually.

ALCOHOL

Though alcohol is a depressant, it is often linked to anxiety. Just one or two drinks can trigger anxiety or a panic attack. But because it usually takes several hours to do so, it may be that the anxiety is a kind of withdrawal, rather than an effect of the alcohol itself. You also have to factor in that anxiety has been linked to alcoholism, and I don't think the cause and effect will ever be neatly understood in terms of which comes first. Complicating matters further, alcohol boosts serotonin levels—but only briefly. This is one more case where the initial positive feelings may lead people to keep doing something that is actually making them feel worse overall. For these reasons, Lovers in trouble should avoid alcohol entirely.

The Lover Diet

To keep your brain chemistry in balance and be the best Lover possible, follow the diet laid out here. The better balanced you are, and the longer you've been in balance, the more your body will be able to handle deviations. But early on, it is advisable to stick closely to the diet. The lists of food choices that come later is not meant to be complete. Rather it just gives you the best and the worst foods for your type. If a particular food in a given category isn't mentioned one way or the other, it is fine to include it.

- 5–7 small meals a day
- 5–7 servings of protein
- 7–11 servings of vegetables
- 2–3 servings of fruit
- 3–5 servings whole grains or whole grain products (note that one serving is just half a cup)

Brain Chemistry Markers

To describe the body's response to stress, be it physical, emotional, or mental, you'd need a list that looks a lot like the symptoms of anxiety—sweating, muscle tension, rapid heartbeats and breathing, and so on. Anxiety is, in fact, just an exaggeration of these ordinary responses.

Anxiety has as many causes as symptoms, or it can occur for no immediately apparent reason. A chemical imbalance in the brain contributes to anxiety, as do psychological factors. It's a bit of a chicken-or-egg situation, however. Does the psychology of a situation cause an overreaction in the brain? Or can an overstimulated brain center create the psychological feelings? In any case, both factors must work together to get a really good case of anxiety going. That's why both drugs and therapy have been effective in treating anxiety—and why natural methods of balancing the brain's physiology are so important.

Anxious people have different brain-wave patterns than do healthy people or people who are depressed. Those findings may help scientists understand anxiety better, but are impractical for diagnosis. More immediately helpful is looking at what we know happens in the brain in times of stress. The brain sends signals to the pituitary and adrenal glands to release

FOOD	BEST CHOICES	GOOD CHOICES	AVOID
Protein (5–7 servings)	Animal: eggs beef lamb dairy products herring yogurt milk cottage cheese halibut chicken turkey salmon Vegetarian: beans (especially lima, navy, garbanzo, black, pinto) nuts (especially cashews, almonds, pistachios, Brazil nuts, hazelnuts, and pecans) seeds (especially sunflower, pumpkin, and sesame) soybeans soy protein products (like tofu) walnuts lentils	Animal: liver and organ meats tuna (canned) Vegetarian: peanuts and peanut butter	shellfish
Vegetables (7–11 servings)	eggplant tomatoes asparagus avocados parsley peas peppers (green and red)	alfalfa sprouts corn mushrooms broccoli Brussels sprouts cabbage carrots cauliflower green leafy vegetables (especially swiss chard, collards,	

FOOD	BEST CHOICES	GOOD CHOICES	AVOID
		mustard greens, kale, and spinach potatoes onions pumpkin sweet potatoes winter squash	
Fruit (2–3 servings)	cherries pineapples plums citrus fruit (especially oranges and grapefruit)	apricots bananas berries (especially strawberries) grapes guava kiwi mangoes melons (especially cantaloupe) papaya	dried fruit fruit juices, except fresh squeezed orange and grapefruit
Whole Grains (3–5 servings)	brown rice corn, stone ground	whole-grain wheat products (including breads and cereals) Whole oats and oatmeal Enriched cereals	white flour white rice pasta (except whole grain pasta)
Sweeteners	maple syrup honey		white sugar chocolate
Beverages	chamomile tea ginseng tea milk	cocoa, sweetened with honey or maple syrup	caffeinated drinks (including coffee, sodas, and diet sodas)
Condiments and Seasonings	brewer's yeast butter cream oils (olive, wheat germ, soybean, corn, sunflower, safflower, sesame, and peanut) (unrefined and cold pressed)		

hormones, specifically adrenaline and noradrenaline. In a crisis, these signals are sent before the cortex (the part of the brain designated to *think* about things) has a chance to weigh in. A lightning-fast response to danger can be critical, so this system is literally a lifesaver when you don't have time to sit around and consider your options. But false alarms—particularly common from a chronically stressed, "burned-out" brain (or a brain on hair-trigger potential after a major trauma)—and the anxiety they create are as problematic as the appropriately functioning system is useful.

There are no specific lab tests for anxiety or panic. But since it is the inappropriate release of these fight-or-flight chemicals that causes anxiety, they can be used as markers if biochemical information is necessary for diagnosis or treatment decisions. But the Lover profile has the least clear biochemical picture of all the types, as you'll see below. If you recognize yourself as the Lover in trouble in this chapter, talk to your doctor about getting your levels of noradrenaline, adrenaline, serotonin, GABA, cortisol, copper, zinc, and magnesium tested. See, "Common Causes of Anxiety and

Normal Levels from Brain Chemistry Markers

Serotonin	55–260 ng/ml (nanograms per milliliter)
Adrenaline	less than 60 pcg/ml (picograms per milliliter)*
Noradrenaline	120–680 pcg/ml**
GABA	0–0.8 micromoles/100 ml (blood test)
	0–10 micromoles/collection (24-hour urine test)
Magnesium	1.3–2.1 meq/L (milliequivalent per liter)
Zinc	60–130 mcg/dl (micrograms per deciliter)
Copper	65–145 mcg/dl

* This is assuming you have your blood test sitting down. If you've been lying down for at least thirty minutes, normal levels are less than 50. If you've been standing at least thirty minutes, normal levels are less than 90.
** As above, this assumes a sitting down blood test. For lying down, the range is 110–410, and for standing the range is 125–700.

Panic" below for other medical issues you should be screened for. You should also look at "The Workup" on page 124 for information on the general tests everyone should have, regardless of their type.

Common Causes of Anxiety and Panic

Several organic factors can cause, exacerbate, or maintain anxiety, and as many as possible should be ruled out before deciding on treatment. These factors include:

Migraines

Copper excess/zinc deficiency

Caffeine

Caffeine withdrawal

Anemia

Hyperthyroidism

Vitamin deficiencies (especially thiamine, vitamin B12, niacin)

Low blood sugar (hypoglycemia)

Withdrawal from alcohol or drugs (particularly depressants, including barbiturates)

Central nervous system stimulants (including amphetamines and cocaine, as well as caffeine)

Sympathomimetic agents, like ephedra

Heavy metal poisoning (especially mercury, arsenic, and lead)

Other psychiatric disorders (including depression, mania, and schizophrenia)

Cardiac conditions

Adrenal dysfunction

Hyperparathyroidism

Vestibular dysfunction

Seizure disorders

Pheochromocytoma

General Medical Screening for Anxiety

To identify other medical conditions causing anxiety and to pinpoint the causes in order to personally tailor the solutions, your doctor should be checking the following:

Complete blood cell count
Electrolytes
Fasting blood sugar levels
Urea
Creatinine
Calcium
Liver panel
Thyroid screen
Urinalysis
Electrocardiogram

NORADRENALINE

Noradrenaline is poorly regulated in people with anxiety who have occasional bursts of excessive activity. High levels of noradrenaline can signify anxiety, with the most consistent results in cases of social phobias. But low levels are often associated with anxiety, too. Some drugs that prevent anxiety do so through the catecholamines, including noradrenaline (and adrenaline).

Since we're talking about Lovers here, it is interesting to note a report that noradrenaline goes up during sexual arousal and declines after orgasm. Although it hasn't been studied, I wonder if some Lovers use sex in an attempt to relieve anxiety (unconscious of the fact that it may temporarily boost neurotransmitters they may be lacking)—or, on the other hand, if Lovers with high noradrenaline are particularly interested in sex.

ADRENALINE

In some cases, adrenaline increases with anxiety, though here again the opposite is sometimes true, too. Adrenaline levels appear to rise during a panic attack. In studies, performance anxiety in particular has been linked to high adrenaline levels. Nearly half of people with a history of panic attacks suffered an attack when *given* adrenaline (many more than in those who were given a placebo), but that's a research technique only, and obviously not a desirable way to get a diagnosis. Studies of patients with social phobias have yielded similar results.

But because results are mixed, it may be that people with anxiety or panic disorders are just more sensitive to the effects of adrenaline—not that their levels are actually any higher. And like noradrenaline, adrenaline facilitates sexual desire, raising some of the same questions as those regarding noradrenaline, discussed above.

SEROTONIN

Serotonin, too, may be high or low in anxiety. Under stress, the brain burns serotonin rapidly, so a state of chronic anxiety can leave levels low. Low serotonin levels may also cause anxiety, panic, and social phobias. The key may be the balance between noradrenaline and serotonin, particularly with panic disorders, so it makes sense to check both levels.

Serotonin acts as a tranquilizer in the brain, so feeling not at all tranquil may indicate a shortage. That's why SSRIs (selective serotonin reuptake inhibitors) are prescribed for anxiety as well as for depression—they can increase serotonin levels in the amygdala. Natural remedies can do the same thing, as you'll see in the Natural Medicine Solutions section below.

GABA (GAMMA-AMINOBUTYRIC ACID)

Many of the common prescription tranquilizers, including the benzodiazepines (the largest-selling drug group in the world, which includes Valium) and barbiturates, work at least in part by boosting the effectiveness of the neurotransmitter GABA (gamma-aminobutyric acid). Some of the options listed in the Natural Medicine Solutions below have the same effect. Low levels of GABA can indicate anxiety, since GABA is the most crucial inhibitory neurotransmitter and lack of it allows some central nervous system reactions to run out of control.

Noradrenaline, adrenaline, and serotonin are more likely to be involved in panic attacks than GABA. So if you have panic attacks, start with tests for those neurotransmitters.

CORTISOL

Cortisol levels are often high in anxiety, and anxious people often show an exaggerated cortisol response. But since cortisol, the "stress hormone," goes up in reaction to any stressor, it isn't a particularly useful marker in identifying anxiety on its own.

COPPER AND ZINC

Copper levels are often high in anxiety, while zinc is often low. As always, the balance between the two is crucial. Lovers who take birth control pills should note that oral contraceptives can lower zinc and raise copper. Again this is only a matter of speculation, but I wonder if Lovers in trouble are any more likely than anyone else to be using birth control pills—or if Lovers are any more likely to give up on birth control because the pills make them feel anxious or exacerbate their anxiety.

MAGNESIUM

Magnesium levels tend to be low in people with anxiety.

Natural Medicine Solutions

The right daily supplements keep your brain chemistry in balance, even when you face the ordinary challenges of life that might otherwise cause stress and/or imbalance, so you can stay your wonderful Lover self. Natural medicine offers solutions, too, if you do get out of balance. Modern medicine offers an array of prescription drug approaches to cure anxiety and panic. Sedatives, tranquilizers, and—the latest twist—antidepressants are among the most frequently prescribed medications aimed at calming people down. The problem is, these drugs come with the risk of addiction, tolerance, and/or overdose. Stopping them can cause rebound effects that are sometimes worse than the condition the patient started out with. The withdrawal process alone can also be worse than whatever the patient began with, even after just a few weeks on synthetic tranquilizers. Or, the drugs might simply not do the trick for you. About 40 percent of patients treated for anxiety with antidepressants don't respond. Another problem with drugs is that they blindly smother symptoms of illness, without treating the cause. Vitamins and herbs, with their beneficial constituents, attempt to correct the cause of the anxiety, an obvious advantage over drugs.

With natural approaches, you can avoid those risks. You may have to try different vitamins, minerals, and herbs before you find the right one, or the right combination, and the right dose for you—though you'd likely have to go through the same experimental phase in settling on a drug treatment, too. This section includes the most promising options.

The supplements listed under "Interventions" are not for daily use over the long term. Rather, they are designed to help you regain balance when you are in trouble. If you are in trouble, they may help as you work to change your diet, and will be more effective still once your diet is under control.

DAILY SUPPLEMENTS

The daily supplements, vitamins, and minerals are powerful on their own, and support the diet. (Their effects will be greatly diminished if not used in conjunction with a balanced diet, however.) As the category implies, you can take them every day indefinitely, though you should take only what you

---

Daily Supplements

Vitamin A: 25,000 IU 5 days a week (natural, from fish liver oil)

B-complex: containing 50–100 mg of each B vitamin

Thiamine (vitamin B1): 100 mg

Pyridoxine (vitamin B6): 50–100 mg

Niacin (vitamin B3): 100–3,000 mg

Vitamin C: 1,000 mg 3–4 times a day

Vitamin E: 200 IU for every twenty years of your life (natural mixed tocopherols)

Calcium: 1,000 mg

Magnesium: 400 mg

need. Where ranges of doses are given, the lower doses are for prevention, while the higher levels are therapeutic for when you are out of balance and/or in trouble. Generally speaking, you should start with lower doses and gradually increase until you experience the desired effect. If you are in trouble right now, you might want to start with a somewhat higher dose.

Vitamin A

Your vitamin A level decreases under stress (or during anxiety), as your body uses it to make the "antistress" adrenal hormones. It helps regulate the dopamine receptors in the brain (and the pituitary gland), so it is crucial to a healthy central nervous system (including, of course, the brain). In fact, vitamin A plays a big role from the very start: it is important in the development of the nervous system of a fetus.

Fatigue, depression, insomnia, and nerve pains in the extremities—as well as anxiety—can be signs of vitamin A deficiency, and supplements can bring relief. The liver stores vitamin A for up to three months, so you don't need a continual daily supplement—in fact, you want to be careful not to get too much vitamin A. That's why you'll often hear the recommendation to take beta-carotene, which the body turns into vitamin A but only as needed.

Take 25,000 IU of natural vitamin A from fish liver oil five days a week, skipping weekends.

Vitamin A

RDA: 5,000 IU

Recommended Dose (general): 10,000 IU

Recommended Dose (in trouble): 25,000 IU

Maximum safe level: Unknown

Contraindications: Don't take vitamin A supplements during pregnancy.

Cod liver oil is so good for you because it is rich in vitamin A. Beef and chicken livers are also good natural sources of vitamin A.

B complex

Deficiencies in the B vitamins, including thiamine, pyridoxine, niacin, riboflavin, folic acid, and cobalamin, have been associated with anxiety. Supplements of B vitamins have been proven to relieve anxiety within three months, as the B vitamins are crucial in helping you feel calm.

If you are not getting enough thiamine, you can experience fearfulness, agitation, emotional instability, insomnia, and psychosomatic complaints. Thiamine helps prevent a racing heartbeat, a common complaint in general anxiety or panic attacks. I usually recommend thiamine supplements of 100 mg a day for anxiety.

Niacin is another B vitamin that is essential in combating anxiety. Regardless of whether or not there is a documented deficiency, niacin supplements have been proven to be as effective as the minor tranquilizers and benzodiazepines used in an animal study. My experience is similar with human patients. A healthy, balanced Lover needs only 100 mg of niacin a day. The Lover in trouble can take progressively higher doses, starting with 100 mg twice a day and increasing up to 1,000 mg three times a day with meals.

The body needs vitamin B6 to make serotonin, so it too is important in controlling anxiety. A deficiency depletes serotonin and can cause anxiety, and supplements (often studied in conjunction with tryptophan) can relieve anxiety. A study of patients who averaged at least two panic attacks per week who were given B6 supplements had no more symptoms after a month, and stayed symptom-free throughout a three-month follow-up period—even if they had discontinued taking the supplements after those first four weeks! I usually recommend 50–100 mg daily. Take the higher dosage if you rarely dream or can't remember your dreams. If you are a heavy dreamer with good dream recall, 50 mg will be enough.

Another good option is a high-dose B-complex supplement, which should cover all the bases and provide a good balance of all the crucial B vitamins.

Vitamin C

Vitamin C, with its sedative effect, can act as a tranquilizer in cases of anxiety; this is a clinical fact. It is also a powerful antioxidant, helping protect the brain and neurons (as well as the rest of the body) from damage from oxygen released during ordinary chemical reactions in the body. Furthermore, as anxiety increases, vitamin C is broken down more rapidly in the body, effectively increasing the body's demand for it.

Vitamin C

RDA: 45 mg

Recommended Dose (general): 1,000–3,000 mg daily

Recommended Dose (in trouble): 1,000–3,000 mg daily; use mineral ascorbate to avoid distention

Maximum safe level: Unknown

Vitamin E

Vitamin E is normally found in the brain and is critical for good mental as well as physical health. It has a calming effect, so it is particularly good for anxious people.

Vitamin E is found in the oils of all grains, nuts, and seeds, but most is lost during processing, since it is destroyed by extremes of temperature (freezing or heating) as well as exposure to air. Simply sitting there for too long can sap most of the vitamin E out of even a rich food source. For such reasons, almost no trace of vitamin E remains in refined oils, flour, or cereals. Cold-pressed vegetable oils (check the label) or virgin olive oil (which means it has been cold-pressed) retain their vitamin E levels. Wheat germ, cottonseed, and safflower oils are (if cold-pressed) excellent sources. Cabbage, spinach, asparagus, and broccoli are among the best vegetables (by vitamin E content). Whole grain wheat, brown rice, and whole oats are also good choices for vitamin E, as are peanuts.

Take 200 IU of natural vitamin E (mixed tocopherols from vegetable oil) each day for every twenty years of your life. That is, if you are under forty, take 200 IU a day; if you are forty or over, take 200 IU twice a day; and if you are sixty or over, take 200 IU three times a day.

Vitamin E

RDA: 10 IU

Recommended Dose (general): 200–600 a day, with meals

Recommended Dose (in trouble): 200–1,000 IU a day, with meals

Maximum safe level: 1,000 IU daily

Contraindications: If you have high blood pressure, overactive thyroid, or heart damage from rheumatic fever, check with your doctor before using vitamin E.

Calcium

Calcium deficiency may show up as anxiety. In fact, the lists of symptoms of an anxiety attack and of mental symptoms of calcium deficiency are very similar. Anxiety related to calcium deficiency is a particularly grouchy, irritable, tense anxiety. Depression, impaired memory, and insomnia are also often along for the ride. Taking calcium is calming and will relieve anxiety.

Calcium

RDA: 1 g (1,000 mg) daily

Recommended Dose (general): 1,000 mg daily

Recommended Dose (in trouble): 1,000–2,000 mg daily

Maximum safe level: Unknown

Contraindications: Consult with a doctor if you have a history of kidney stone formation.

Calcium also lowers histamine, which is no doubt how it works in high-histamine anxiety. In addition, rapid breathing (like the hyperventilation common in anxiety) lowers the level of calcium in the bloodstream, which can cause a calcium deficiency, leading to confusion, dizziness, numbness, and muscle cramps.

Dairy products are already famous as sources of calcium, but green leafy vegetables, peas, beans, potatoes, cauliflower, and molasses are also good sources. Certain mineral waters also provide calcium in the diet, and an increasing number of products are fortified with this mineral.

Take 1,000 mg a day of calcium citrate, lactate or gluconate. Liquid forms are recommended for easier absorption, and you should look for formulas mixed with magnesium, as the two minerals are crucial to each other's performance.

Magnesium

Magnesium deficiency has also been associated with anxiety, especially nervousness and sleeping problems. Magnesium also helps to control a racing heartbeat. Magnesium supplements (I generally recommend 400–600 mg a day) have been shown to relieve anxiety and are often given together with calcium. Magnesium is best known as a remedy for insomnia, though it has many other general medicine uses, besides being good for depression. Studies show that not only do almost all patients fall asleep faster, enjoy uninterrupted sleep, and wake up refreshed, but they also experience less tension and anxiety during the day.

Magnesium

RDA: 6 mg daily

Recommended Dose (general): 400 mg daily

Recommended Dose (in trouble): 600 mg daily

Maximum safe level: Unknown

Contraindications: Low blood pressure

INTERVENTIONS—FOR TIMES OF TROUBLE ONLY

Lovers have many natural options for interventions. When it comes to herbs, try one at a time, preferably at least for a while before you combine them. For information on using natural and prescription items together, see p. 102.

INTERVENTION	DAILY DOSE
Amino Acids	
Tryptophan	1–9 g a day (500–1,500 mg at bedtime for insomnia)
5-HTP	100 mg 1–3 times a day
Glutamine	500 mg 4 times a day
Herbs	
Kava	70 mg 1–3 times a day
Valerian	3–4 cups of tea a day
Chamomile	3–4 cups of tea a day
Passionflower	1–2 cups of tea a day
St. John's wort	300 mg (0.3 percent hypericin) 1–4 times a day
Ginseng	3–4 cups of tea a day

Tryptophan or 5-HTP (5-Hydroxy-Tryptophan)

Because it, too, can increase serotonin, either tryptophan or 5-HTP may be a good choice in some cases of anxiety. In fact, tryptophan performed as

---

5-HTP

Recommended dose (in trouble): 100–300 mg daily

Maximum safe level: Unknown. As with tryptophan, there is a theoretical (but extremely rare) risk of serotonin syndrome. If 5-HTP raises serotonin too high, the result can be confusion, fever, shivering, sweating, diarrhea, muscle spasms, and, very rarely, death.

Contraindications: Do not drive or operate heavy machinery until you're familiar with how 5-HTP affects you, and whether it makes you drowsy. Do not take it with psychiatric drugs without consulting the prescribing physician.

Tryptophan

Recommended dose (in trouble): 1–9 g daily (500–1,500 mg at bedtime for insomnia)

Maximum safe level: Unknown. Don't exceed 3 grams a day unless you are under a doctor's close supervision. Theoretically, if L-tryptophan raises serotonin too high, serotonin syndrome can result, characterized by confusion, fever, shivering, sweating, diarrhea, muscle spasms, and, very rarely, death.

Contraindications: Don't drive or operate heavy machinery until you're familiar with how tryptophan affects you, and whether it makes you drowsy. Don't take it with an antidepressant drug without discussing it with your doctor first.

well as prescription drugs in one study of anxiety disorders. Agoraphobia and panic attacks most commonly seem to involve low serotonin levels, so tryptophan may be most likely to be effective in those cases.

L-glutamine

In the brain, glutamine is converted into GABA (gamma-aminobutyric acid), a natural tranquilizer. In anxiety, insufficient levels of glutamine may be available and/or insufficient levels of GABA may be manufactured. The amino acid L-glutamine is calming because it is converted into glutamic acid, which is used to make GABA. Glutamine fights depression, fatigue, and pain, in addition to having tranquilizing effects.

L-glutamine

Recommended dose (in trouble): 500 mg 4 times a day

Maximum safe level: Unknown

Contraindications: None

Kava

Kava, sometimes known as kava kava, is made from the root of a South Pacific pepper tree and is widely used as a social and ceremonial beverage in the Pacific Islands. Kava is so widely used, in fact, that it is easy to believe it is responsible for the relaxed, laid-back atmosphere of the Islands. Kava is now sold around the world in prepackaged forms as a remedy for anxiety, stress, and insomnia. Its calming effect makes it an excellent sedative, and studies have proven it to be as effective as prescription tranquilizers for mild to moderate anxiety. Yet kava comes with none of the sedation, lethargy, drowsiness, memory impairment, diminished concentration, fuzziness of thinking, delayed reaction times, or threat of addiction that can accompany the common antianxiety drugs.

Kava enhances the work of GABA, thereby helping reduce anxiety. The herb also limits the activity of dopamine, and one theory holds that it calms an overactive amygdala.

There is good evidence that kava works against anxiety (and insomnia), and the same studies show no tolerance, dependence, or withdrawal symptoms, which are common with prescription tranquilizers. Several studies

---

Kava

Recommended dose (in trouble): 70–210 mg kavalactones daily for anxiety; or 150–200 mg daily before bed for insomnia

Maximum safe level: Unknown

Contraindications: Don't take with alcohol, barbiturates, antidepressants, benzodiazepines, or other tranquilizers or sleeping pills, anticoagulants or antiplatelet agents (including aspirin), antipsychotics, drugs for treating Parkinson's disease, or drugs that depress the central nervous system. Using kava can exacerbate Parkinson's disease, increasing muscular weakness and twitching, and so it is to be avoided. Don't take during pregnancy or while breastfeeding.

have taught us that kava can outperform placebo by the end of four to eight weeks (though it may take four weeks before effectiveness is felt). Even studies of patients with moderate to severe anxiety revealed the benefits of kava in all the major categories of anxiety, including agoraphobia, generalized anxiety disorder, specific phobia, and social phobia. More than half of the patients in the group taking kava in a twenty-four-week study were "very improved" on standard scales of anxiety, fear, and tension, and the rate of insomnia decreased markedly, too. (The other comparison group, which was taking a placebo, didn't fare as well.) Side effects were rare but appeared at the same rate in those taking kava and those on placebo. Animal studies have proven that kava can induce sleep and also that it produces muscle relaxation.

Germany's Commission E (like our FDA) approves kava for "nervous anxiety, stress, and restlessness," recommending 70 mg two or three times a day (or 180–210 mg one hour before bed for insomnia). Most studies use kava extract standardized to 70 percent kavalactones (the active ingredient), with 100 mg kava (and so 70 mg kavalactones) given three times a day. However, that concentration is not available over the counter in the United States. Instead, you'll most likely be faced with a bit of a math problem: How many pills (usually between 100 and 250 mg each) you need to get the equivalent of 70 mg kavalactones depends on the percentage of kavalactones, which ranges upward from 30 percent.

Start by taking 70–85 mg kavalactones once a day in the evening. If that doesn't do it for you (allow yourself at least a week to find out), add another dose in the morning and stick with that for at least a week before adding a third dose, midday, if you need it. You should talk with your doctor about any medication you are taking, including herbs and supplements, but be sure to do so before taking more than the 210 mg kavalactones a day. Once you've calmed down, cut out one dose every few days.

Kava is available in capsules or as a liquid. Take particular care when driving while using kava until you are experienced with exactly how it affects you.

Some people may have an allergic reaction to kava and should obviously avoid using it. And extremely high doses over many months can bring complications, particularly skin problems, though they generally clear up when you stop taking the herb.

Valerian

The antianxiety herb Valerian is a mild tranquilizer, sedative, calmative, and muscle relaxant. It is used for nervousness, insomnia and other sleeping problems, restlessness, tension, lack of concentration, excitability, stress, hysteria, agitation, and angst—many of which are problems for a Lover in trouble. The biggest-selling prescription tranquilizer, Valium, is derived from valerian.

Valerian is an important herb in both Ayurveda (the root comes from east India) and traditional Chinese medicine and was widely used in this country before synthetic drugs became available around World War I. It has been safely used as a remedy for anxiety and sleep problems for at least a thousand years. Now we understand that it works (just as benzodiazepine tranquilizers do) by boosting the neurotransmitter GABA, which has sedative properties, and many clinical studies have proven its effectiveness. It has even been studied for very specific types of anxiety, including performance anxiety and driving in heavy traffic, and has been shown to work across the board.

Valerian is available in capsules, tablets, tinctures, and extracts, and can also be taken as a tea or even added to bath water and absorbed through the skin. Most extracts are standardized to 0.8 percent valeric acids. Larger

---

Valerian

Recommended Dose (in trouble): 3–4 cups of tea a day
　　　　　　　　　　　　(for insomnia): 1–2 cups of tea at bedtime

Maximum safe level: Unknown

Contraindications: Do not take valerian with alcohol, phenobarbital, or benzodiazepines.

doses taken at bedtime, rather than spread throughout the day, are recommended for insomnia.

Unlike many similarly used prescription drugs, valerian is not addictive. It is actually helpful for withdrawal from tranquilizers or sleeping pills, though you should work with a doctor's supervision to do that, especially since you may require somewhat larger doses than usual.

Valerian sometimes, though rarely, *causes* nervousness, and obviously anyone who experiences that side effect should choose a different approach.

Chamomile

The flavonoids and essential oils in chamomile are what make this sedative herb powerful. It soothes anxiety or can be used preventively. Some have called it the European equivalent of ginseng—it is good for whatever ails you, as a sort of general tonic. It makes a relaxing tea, which is often helpful for sleeping difficulties.

Anyone allergic to ragweed, asters, chrysanthemums, or other Asteraceae family members should avoid the closely related chamomile.

Chamomile

Recommended dose (in trouble): 3–4 cups of tea a day

Maximum safe level: Unknown

Contraindications: If you are allergic to ragweed, chrysanthemums, and other daisies, you may want to avoid chamomile, which is in the same family. (You won't necessarily be sensitive to it, though, so it may be worth a try.)

Passionflower

The natural tranquilizer passionflower is extremely popular in Europe as a sedative, most commonly given for anxiety, irritability, and insomnia. In fact, it is the most popular choice in England. Germany's Commission E approves it for "nervous unrest."

Passionflower extracts are often sold standardized to 3.5–4 percent isovi-

> **Passionflower**
>
> **Recommended dose (in trouble):** 1–2 cups of tea at bedtime
>
> **Maximum safe level:** Unknown
>
> **Contraindications:** None

texin, a powerful flavonoid, and looking for that on the label helps ensure you're getting a constant level of the active ingredient.

I recommend taking passionflower as a tea from the dried plant.

St. John's Wort (Hypericum)

St. John's wort works for anxiety as well as depression when low serotonin level is the issue. A mild sedative and natural tranquilizer, it may bind to the same receptors as benzodiazepines.

> **St. John's Wort**
>
> **Recommended dose (in trouble):** 300 mg (0.3 percent hypericin) 1–4 times a day
>
> **Maximum safe level:** 1,200 mg daily. (Above that, there's no additional benefit anyway.)
>
> **Contraindications:** St. John's wort increases sensitivity to sunlight, and fair-skinned people especially should watch their exposure. Do not take St. John's wort with MAO inhibitors (or for four weeks after stopping them), coumidin, Digoxin, protease inhibitors and indinavir (for HIV), cyclosporine (for cancer), or photosensitizing drugs including tetracycline. Do not take it while on drugs following an organ transplant. This herb is not for pregnant or nursing women. It can speed up the breakdown of (interfering with the effectiveness of) prescription medication, including blood thinners, cholesterol-lowering medications, seizure medications, cancer medications, drugs used to fight HIV, drugs that prevent organ transplant rejection, and birth control pills.

Ginseng

Panax ginseng and Siberian ginseng are nerve tonics. That is, they are good for the nervous system in general. Ginseng can raise noradrenaline levels, which obviously wouldn't be helpful in cases where high noradrenaline is causing anxiety. It would be helpful, however, if low noradrenaline is the problem. But ginseng may also raise cortisol, which might be counterproductive if cortisol is already high. Because ginseng is an adaptogen, meaning it has potentially opposite effects on the body, and your body gets whichever it needs, it may be helpful for mild anxiety even though in some people it is a stimulant. Because adrenal gland tissue, like brain tissue, is neuroendocrine tissue, ginseng provides adrenal support along with brain nourishment. Siberian ginseng is supposed to be particularly supportive for overtaxed adrenal glands.

A natural tranquilizer and stimulant, ginseng root contains concentrated stores of vitamins and minerals. The nourishment of our nerves is experienced as a rush of good feelings replacing our uneasy anxiety about twenty minutes after sipping a cup of ginseng tea. Anxiety, like depression, is one way the brain has of expressing that it is malnourished. These negative states only exist in a malnourished brain.

Chinese and Russian ginseng are reputed to be the most potent, trailed by Korean ginseng. American ginseng is the mildest. The more potent the ginseng, the more expensive it is.

Ginseng

Recommended dose (in trouble): 3–4 cups of tea a day

Maximum safe level: Unknown

Contraindications: Don't take ginseng if you have severe anxiety, manic depression, heart palpitations, asthma, or emphysema. This herb is not for use during pregnancy. Do not use it at the same time as caffeine, ephedra, or other stimulants if you have high blood pressure or migraines or if you are sick.

Mind/Body and Lifestyle Changes

Anxiety is not necessarily a negative. As a warning of external or internal stress, it can save your life. Lovers are taking advantage of an excellent self-defense system. But when those signals run amok, the results can be devastating. When that happens, your first stop should be proper nutrition. For many people, all they need to do to remove any biochemical cause of anxiety is to stop eating junk food and dine instead on whole, healthy, unrefined foods, and use the supplements that are right for them. A few other basic lifestyle choices, along with avoiding sugar, caffeine, and alcohol, as explained earlier, may be necessary for the best biochemical balance.

SMOKING

Smoking may be a habit acquired or maintained to handle anxiety. But nicotine can cause or exacerbate anxiety—even secondhand smoke can be a problem. And whether or not smoking makes you anxious, *stopping* smoking surely can. We all know by now that it's the healthy thing to do, but if fear of the withdrawal effects is what's stopping you from quitting, take heart: The same natural solutions for any kind of anxiety can help you quit. St. John's wort and valerian are particularly helpful in taking the edge off as you cut back and eliminate smoking.

DRUGS

We've already covered the problems with caffeine in the Dietary Guidelines section, but other central nervous system stimulants—heavy hitters like cocaine and amphetamines—can also cause devastating anxiety and must be avoided. Lovers are especially likely to experience that effect. Many anxious people use various kinds of drugs in an attempt (whether or not they are doing it on purpose) to control their symptoms, but most—including painkillers, tranquilizers, cocaine, and amphetamines—not only won't work, they'll actually intensify the anxiety.

ADDICTION

Lovers in trouble are prone to various addictions, such as sugar, caffeine, alcohol, cigarettes, overeating, drugs (prescription or illegal), and even nervous habits. Those things appear at first to soothe anxious feelings, though they in fact almost invariably make them worse overall. Breaking addictions—though the process itself can cause anxiety—is an important part of regaining and maintaining biochemical balance in the brain.

Sooner or later, all addictions interfere with good nutrition, through loss of appetite or the direct interference with stomach absorption of nutrients or creation of deficiencies. Overcoming the addiction itself will have an immediately beneficial effect on the nutrition of your brain chemistry.

Nutrition for Quitting an Addiction

If you are ready to quit smoking, drinking, or any other addiction, these nutrients will help minimize the withdrawal symptoms:

L-glutamine: 500 mg, 4 times a day

Vitamin C: 1,000 mg 6 times daily for the first two or three days, tapering off to 1–3 g a day

Niacin (vitamin B3): 1,000 mg, six times daily for the first two or three days, tapering off to 1–3 g a day

Eat a small, high-protein snack every hour you are awake for the first two or three days; then, taper off to a single high-protein snack a day for two to three weeks.

After a few days, the vitamin C and niacin can be reduced to 1–2 grams daily.

The L-glutamine can be stopped after 2–3 weeks.

EXERCISE

Exercise is often recommended as an antidote for depression, but it is equally effective at fighting anxiety. It lifts serotonin and also, to a lesser degree, noradrenaline. The noradrenaline will recede as soon as you are no longer active, while serotonin remains high. With gentle exercise, like stretching, walking, yoga, tai chi, qi gong, or low-impact aerobics, you'll get the serotonin boost without affecting noradrenaline.

TALK THERAPY

For Lovers, insight-oriented psychotherapy, meditation, or any introspective method can help them understand any emotional or psychological factors in their anxiety. Lovers, openly emotional as they are, are quite *good* at psychotherapy. Since the therapeutic relationship is usually fairly intense, it's a natural for a Lover. The choice of a therapist is an important one for anyone, but never more so than for Lovers, because of the tremendous stock they place in relationships.

Lovers in trouble need to bolster their self-confidence, or they'll run the risk of repeating bad relationships. They are often following a template they learned in childhood. As adults they may get involved with rejecting partners over and over again because that is all they've known. The "insight" many are after in insight-oriented therapy is this pattern and its deepest roots. Just identifying it helps to avoid it in the future, but you can't avoid it if you can't recognize it.

Another common discovery for Lovers engaging in intense introspection is the way their use of deception causes anxiety. This may be in the form of some conflict they've repressed (in effect, lying to themselves)—such as staying in an abusive relationship or denying earlier abuse. Or it may be that their deception of others is rebounding to themselves in ways they didn't foresee. For example, if they lead a partner to believe that they are not looking for a commitment as a way to get a foot in the door but they are really marriage-minded, that relationship is bound to cause heartache.

Lovers may also get good results from cognitive-behavioral therapy. Cognitive therapy, as it is sometimes known, is goal-oriented therapy using practical strategies, usually over the short term. The therapist acts as coach and teacher, explaining what is known about the patient's issues and suggesting concrete steps to resolve them. The patient then practices those techniques outside of therapy sessions. It is designed to help you identify the thoughts and perceptions making you anxious, and where and how they may be exaggerated. The idea is to learn to accurately assess your situation without overoptimism and without constantly jumping to worst-case scenarios.

There are several avenues that Lovers usually benefit from exploring, whether on their own or with a therapist. (Lovers tend to be good at working *with* someone, as long as he or she is the right "someone.") The most important thing may be withdrawing from their overinvestment in relationships with others. Discovering and developing their own autonomy should be a prerequisite for Lovers contemplating a relationship. This is easier said than done, as Lovers feel so compelled to be in relationships. The key is finding their authentic selves—not the "self" they've molded themselves into to fit into one relationship or another—and respecting themselves and their own desires. From that position, a Lover can finally participate in a relationship as a fully empowered individual.

TRY IT, YOU'LL LIKE IT

The simplest exercise I recommend to Lovers is just this: remember to breathe. To calm down quickly and easily, try a series of five to fifteen long, slow inhalations and exhalations of clean air through your nostrils with your mouth closed.

As a Lover, you'll also benefit from stretching out the aspects of your personality that resemble your opposite type (the Dreamer—see pie chart on p. 28) as well as your adjoining types.

Try staying home, alone, one night—and just sit and think. Don't have anyone over, don't make phone calls, don't put your TV or radio on for company. Experience what it is like to just be yourself, by yourself.

You can also focus on *not* flirting the next time you are out. If you are on a date, be attentive to your date only, and only politely interested in anyone else you meet while you are out. I'm not saying you usually are scanning the room for better offers or looking to ditch your date at the slightest provocation, but many Lovers have a tendency to flirt with the waiter, bartender, ticket taker, cabdriver, and anyone else who crosses their path. Not that there is generally any harm in that, but it should be interesting for you to observe what it feels like *not* to.

Lovers can also find new balance within themselves by balancing their effortless abilities in "soft" social skills with learning a new practical "hard" skill, like sewing, pottery, or accounting.

9

The
Brain
Chemistry
Diet

Each of the preceding chapters gives diet advice tailored to each of six character types. Those guidelines are most important when reestablishing biochemical balance within the brain but are not necessarily needed simply to maintain good physical and mental health. No matter what rules you're following, each person will have individual concerns—and tastes—to satisfy. But there are a handful of general rules of healthy eating that apply to everyone, which we will explore here.

I'm not flogging any trendy set of dietary laws here, so I'm sure to rile devotees of the latest thing "everybody's" doing—whatever it may be this season. I'm not anti-fat. Or anti-carb. Or anti-protein. You need all of those in combination (and reasonable proportion) for good health. I *am* an advocate of moderation in all things (including moderation!).

The high-protein, limited-carbohydrate 5–7-meals-a-day program recommended so frequently throughout this book is primarily an acute healing diet and generally is not necessary once you are in good shape, biochemically speaking. I recommend that diet to my patients nine out of ten times, I'd say, since the problems they bring to me are so commonly the result of poor nutrition. (I do *not*, however, recommend it to someone who has kidney damage or who is obese, for example.)

Once you're back on track, having corrected any imbalances, what the right diet can do for you is to keep you in good shape, allow you to manage stresses of all kinds, and help you stay mentally sharp. Beyond moderation in all things, I'm just reaffirming well-established principles of the highest-quality nutrition. To optimize your physical well-being—including the well-being of your brain, thoughts, emotions, and moods—you need just four basic guidelines: eat a rich variety of natural foods; choose fresh, whole foods that are as close as possible to their natural state; opt for clean foods, using organic and free-range items whenever possible; and, get a good amount of healthy fats and oils, but strictly limit saturated and trans-fatty acids.

Eat a Rich Variety of Natural Foods

A rich variety of natural foods includes some meats, fish, and dairy (that is, for people who don't have specific objections to animal products), but the bulk of almost everyone's choices over the long term should come from vegetables, fruits, legumes, and whole grains. Eating a variety of these nutrient-dense foods is the most efficient way to ensure that you get sufficient quantities of a wide range of vitamins and minerals, as well as the other micronutrients and phytochemicals that are proving to be equally important to good health. For most people, this means you're going to be getting more than the five servings per day that the government has been tirelessly recommending. Vegetables, fruits, legumes, and whole grains are also generally low in fat, usually between 0.5 and 2 percent. Furthermore, the fats they do have are almost always the healthy kind. They are also almost always low in calories and high in fiber. If your plate is always mostly full of foods from these categories, you'll stay slim as well as fit.

A vegetarian diet is richer in nutrients than the average American diet, and it can be lower in fat (though it can certainly also be high in fat). But unless you abstain for personal or philosophical reasons, meat can be a healthy part of your diet. It is a natural food and very nutrient-dense.

If your diet is relatively high in protein—especially animal protein, meaning it is also higher in fat—you may need to exercise more to compensate. (Or, to put it another way, those who exercise more may use more protein and fat healthfully.) The main problem with animal protein is that it is digested slowly. It stays in the intestinal tract a long time, giving the body more time to absorb any toxins in the fat and giving the toxins more time to affect the body. Vegetable protein, on the other hand, digests quickly, and all the roughage (fiber) sweeps the intestinal tract like a broom.

Choose Fresh, Whole Foods That Are as Close as Possible to Their Natural State

Here's your new diet mantra: get the whites out.

Get rid of white sugar, white flour, white rice, and white oils. These highly refined, processed foods are largely stripped of any nutritional value in the bargain. For example, 80 percent of minerals are lost by refining or canning. And that's just the first part of the problem. Digestion rapidly breaks these simple carbohydrates down into sugars, which are empty calories that tax the body's reserves while contributing nothing of value. Yet these "whites" are the dominant ingredient in the average American diet. No wonder so many of us are malnourished, tired, stressed, sick, and just plain not feeling our best.

So choose whole grains, including whole grain bread and pasta, and brown rice. Avoid all refined, canned, and frozen food. The less processed your food is, the better. Avoid eating things manufactured by humans, opting instead for the handiwork of Mother Nature, in as close to their original state as possible.

Choose fresh foods, as close to harvest as possible. Eat what is in season. Be wary of foods grown in distant parts of the world and shipped by air. As often as possible, select locally grown produce. For all kinds of food, buy the freshest stuff you can find and eat it as soon as possible after purchase. Cook and eat meat, for example, on the same day you buy it. Buy smaller quantities of everything, so food doesn't sit around the house, deteriorating in quality and tempting you to overeat.

Aim to eat much of your food raw, but cook anything that common sense tells you should be cooked, like meat, fish, grains, legumes, and eggs. Cooking meat and fish removes fat and blood and kills bacteria and parasites. Eggs may harbor viruses that cooking destroys, and an antivitamin in the white of the egg destroys the yolk's biotin unless the egg-white is cooked. The minerals that grains contain are for the most part available to the human body only once they've been released by cooking. The minerals in raw beans and grains are bound to substances called phytates that can prevent mineral absorption.

For most fruits and many vegetables (including most of the salad vegetables), raw is better. Many vitamins, including vitamin C and all the B-complex vitamins, are destroyed by heat and light (one reason it is good to refrigerate your food). One exception is the cabbage family, which contains both harmful phytates and thyroid-inhibiting compounds that are destroyed by heat—so they should be cooked. That's not to say you should never have cabbage raw—nor should you forgo cooked vegetables of other kinds all the time. Just make sure that your other food choices are the most nutrient-rich they can be. When you do cook vegetables, steaming is the way to go. Keep them out of the cooking water, which leaches nutrients right out.

Through heavy use of refined (white) sugar, humans have managed to separate sweetness from goodness—qualities that come paired in nature. Unlike refined sugars, which do your body no favors, *natural* sugars like honey, maple syrup, molasses, fruit, and whole sugar cane, are actually beneficial. They contain the nutrients our bodies need to metabolize sugars.

In addition to following the fats/oils guidelines (see p. 329), make an effort to avoid all "white" oils. That covers most of the "supermarket" oils, which are commercially processed at intense heat—literally boiling them to death and stripping them of vital nutrients. Look for oils like olive oil and sesame oil, whose rich colors are your first clue that their nutrients are still intact. Virgin or extra-virgin olive oil is less refined and therefore the best. Check the label for "100% virgin, cold pressed."

The nutrient-stripping that occurs during food refinement is well documented. The existing solution to the vitamin deficiencies caused by processing has been to "enrich" foods by adding back in just a few vitamins and ignoring the rest of the known nutrients. (In the case of white flour, en-

Keep It in the Dark

Light can destroy nutrients in oils just as heat can, so it is best to buy oil in cans, which keep it in the dark. Dark glass is a good runner-up. Whatever the material, buy it in small containers, and use up the oil promptly to be sure it is fresh when you eat it. Also, be sure to store oil in a cool, dark place.

richment entails just four vitamins, compared to the thirty identified nutrients found in unrefined flour.) And enriching foods can cause problems of its own. For example, vitamin D added to milk can interfere with magnesium absorption (ironically, the D is added in part because it is crucial for making use of the calcium in milk—*as is magnesium*).

To whatever extent is possible, eat food you've prepared yourself (or had prepared specially for you). Unless you're cooking, you can't know exactly what you're eating. Most restaurants use additives and previously prepared food. As with all of these rules I'm setting out, there are times you will just have to do whatever you have to do in the course of your day, even if optimal nutrition isn't at the top of the priority list. The best thing to do is not to worry about imperfections—the worry will kill you faster than a trip to a fast-food joint will.

Your car doesn't run on gasoline alone. You also need to put in oil, coolant, and a battery. If you try to live on white flour and white sugar, it's like putting in gas but never adding oil, water, and fluids—sooner or later the car will break down. The human body is that much more complicated in its need for the correct nutrients. Optimal health is the result of many, many chemical reactions within the body. All nutrients have to be present for those reactions to occur optimally. Nature has placed everything together in convenient packages, and when we choose whole natural foods as our fuel, we automatically get everything we need. But for reasons of convenience or taste, more often than not those nutrients are separated out (refined), and major portions of essential ingredients are lost. When we try to improve on Mother Nature, rather than making things better, we make them worse. Even if we keep running, the long-term damage to the engine is very real.

Opt for Clean Foods, Using Organic and Free-Range Items Whenever Possible

Most of what Americans eat is grown with pesticides, and traces remain on the food when you bring it home. (Pesticides also contaminate our soil, water, and air, but that's a story for another day.) The risks of malnutrition are much greater than the risks from pesticides, so everyone needs to partake of vegetables, fruits, and grains regardless of how they are grown. But buying organic ensures that you get no pesticides, and it supports farmers using environmentally sound practices and hopefully using non-genetically modified seeds. When you can't buy organic, thoroughly wash your produce with a spray hose and/or a scrub brush, and peel anything you can. Peeling is especially important for anything waxed, like apples or cucumbers, as the wax seals in the pesticides, so they can't be washed or rubbed off. The peel is often the most nutritious part, however, and so with organic you don't have to make any trade-offs.

Look for organic and "free range" or "range fed" meat, chicken, eggs, milk, and other dairy products to avoid the antibiotics, hormones, tenderizers, and pesticides contaminating the factory-farmed versions of those foods. Ideally, you can also buy products from animals raised on organically grown food.

In addition, standard factory farming pens animals up, so they don't get any exercise, building up the fat in the meat. That's as unhealthy for us as it is for them. We all know by now we should trim the visible fat from meat because of the saturated fat it puts in our bodies. Remember, too, that fat is where the chemicals that can't be metabolized by the liver are stored.

You should also avoid consuming the blood of an animal because it carries the hormones (both what's fed to the animals to make them grow freakishly fast and the stress hormones that flood an animal's body at the slaughter). The longer you cook meat, the more blood and fat you'll lose. It also helps to cook meat raised above the heat or pan to allow the blood and fat to drip off.

Kosher meat is a good choice, if you can find it, as the animals aren't treated with hormones and are inspected to make sure they are healthy. Further, because the rabbi recites a special prayer over the animal, which is said to calm it, before its throat is quietly slit, the animal is tranquil at the time of its death instead of terrified and filled with adrenaline. The blood is drained from the meat, so you can avoid ingesting the stress hormones that might nonetheless flood an animal's body at slaughter. The meat is also salted and then rinsed and soaked in cold water. Salt is antibacterial and an excellent solvent, drawing out the blood from the meat just as it draws out a wine stain from a rug. Water is also a good solvent, bringing out more blood and fat, and the combination leaves the koshered meat less likely to be contaminated with bacteria, hormones, and other potentially harmful substances.

Fish is generally healthy, as I've said, but you do have to exercise some caution. Think small. The bigger the fish, the more concentrated the levels of any toxins will be. Sardines are cleaner than tuna, for example, and salmon falls somewhere in between. Studies indicate that having two or three servings of fish a week can cut your risk of heart disease in half—just choose your fish wisely. I recommend both fresh- and saltwater fish, though saltwater fish does have the advantage of providing the mineral iodine, a necessary nutrient that is especially important for preventing hypothyroidism.

Get a Good Amount of Healthy Fats and Oils, but Strictly Limit Saturated Fats and Trans-Fatty Acids

Make sure your diet is low in fat, as a lowfat diet is good for longevity. Excesses of saturated fats (animal fats) in particular contribute to heart disease, breast cancer, and colon cancer, among other serious health concerns. Even worse are partially hydrogenated oils—cheap solid or semi-solid vegetable fats used widely in prepared foods because they don't turn rancid for a long time. Besides being a processed (not fresh or natural) food, hydrogenated and partially hydrogenated fats and oils contain up to 25 percent trans-fatty acids. Trans-fatty acids, or partially hydrogenated oils, increase "bad" cholesterol levels and decrease "good" cholesterol, even though they may start out as healthy fats before they are hydrogenated.

But fat is not always the enemy. You need certain healthy fats in your diet for smooth functioning of your body. Healthy fats are the secret of the "Mediterranean diet," which is famous for gourmet food and for promoting longevity—lots of healthy olive oil and fish to complement plenty of fresh veggies, grains, and small (by American standards) servings of meat and dairy.

Monounsaturated olive oil and canola oil are wise choices. They are more stable than polyunsaturated vegetable oils like corn, safflower, and sunflower, so they don't break down (a politer way of saying get rancid) as quickly, and they don't release as many of the cancer- and heart-disease–causing free radicals. Polyunsaturated oils, eaten fresh, are a reasonable second choice. You also need fat-soluble vitamins (A, D, E, and K)—and the fats that contain them and/or help your body to retain them.

Essential fatty acids (EFAs) are an important category of healthy fats. They are needed for the healthy growth and functioning of every cell in the body, but our bodies cannot manufacture them—we must get them from our diets. Modest amounts of EFAs are found in most oils and fats. Particularly rich sources include raw linseed and cod liver oils. One teaspoonful per day provides your daily needs. Corn, safflower, and sunflower seed oils have fewer EFAs, so you'd need one tablespoon of those to meet your requirements.

Omega-3 oils, mainly fish oils, though they are sometimes derived from algae and plankton, are used to build brain cells and transmit impulses from one brain cell to the next. (Alpha-linolenic acid is the name of omega-3 fats from land-based sources, like soybeans.) Omega-3 EFAs are especially highly concentrated in brain cell membranes, particularly in the cortex, the outer brain center of higher thinking. We need healthy amounts to think and to use our memories. Omega-3s also thin the blood and so help the brain cells by allowing better circulation, which means more oxygen and nutrients carried to the brain cells. Omega-3s also help us handle stress.

The omega-6 oils (linoleic acid), derived primarily from vegetable oils in plants and seeds, such as flaxseed oil, are the most abundant EFAs, and offer similar benefits. They are an extremely beneficial addition to the diet.

No matter which oil you are using, be sure to buy it as fresh as possible. Store it in the refrigerator to maximize freshness. Omega-3 fats can be destroyed by heat, light, and even air (oxygen), so keep them in a cool, dark place. Dark bottles are best. Buy cold-pressed oils to make sure the nutrients haven't been destroyed in processing.

Dairy fat also has benefits, so as both a butter lover and a physician, I do *not* endorse the nonfat dairy product mandate. Besides being a good source of fat-soluble vitamins, dairy fat has antitumor, antiviral, and antibiotic

Good Sources of Omega-3 Oils

Oils:	Fish:
olive	salmon
corn	mackerel
flaxseed (linseed)	trout
pumpkin	sardines
wheat germ	tuna (bluefin)
canola (rapeseed)	eel
soybean	roe
walnut	herring
fish	sablefish
	whitefish
	turbot
Meat and Poultry:	shark
lamb	bluefish
chicken liver	bass
eggs (the yolk is a good source	smelt
of both omega-3 and omega-6	swordfish
essential fats)	oysters and other shellfish

factors. Nonfat and lowfat dairy products are lacking in all these vital nutrients, and have a lot of additives (and so not as much milk) that your body doesn't need. That's on top of their taste appeal. Cats won't drink skim milk. And I, for one, can't blame them.

Furthermore, fat makes food taste good. On top of that, a little fat gives a sense of satisfaction, a satiety factor, that actually helps you eat fewer calories overall. Better you should get the fat—and the nutrients that come with it—than miss out on healthy foods altogether because you find them unappealing.

While I'm on the subject of dairy fat, let me address the old butter vs. margarine debate. I'd choose real butter every time. Butter is a natural food that has been in use since the dawn of history, while margarine is a twentieth-century synthetically processed food. Margarine is made by the hydrogenation of polyunsaturated liquid corn or soybean oil, converting it into the solid saturated fat. Worse, trans-fats, which have lost their EFA activity, are formed during hydrogenation, and the high temperature destroys the fat-soluble vitamins A and E, along with other nutrients.

In reality, you don't even need to know the four basic guidelines described above to eat healthfully. The single piece of advice you need to keep in mind is this—*think natural.*

Changing the way you eat will not be easy at first. Each character type has particular eating strategies best for their brain chemistry. And each type has favored foods that may get them into trouble. Unfortunately, we tend to love what is bad for us, so we all need to moderate some things we tend to overindulge in. We need to develop some self-restraint, and we may need to discover some new foods, or new ways of eating.

If you're diligent for just one month, I promise you smooth sailing thereafter. Four weeks is long enough to create and cement new habits, so you'll no longer need your "old ways" just because you don't know what else to do. And in that short time, you'll notice a dramatic difference in the way you think and feel—and once you've had that, you won't *want* to go back. Finally, once you've gotten your body well nourished, you'll be able to "cheat"

Take Everything You Read about Salt with . . . a Grain of Salt

Salt is the victim of too much bad press. Sky-high levels surely are not good for the human body, and the connection between excess sodium and high blood pressure (and the attendant risk of heart disease) is well established. But all the negative attention has over-shadowed the fact that you can suffer from *insufficient* salt. Salt is an absolute basic essential in the bloodstream. And while salt won't kill *us,* as long as we keep it reasonable, it does kill a lot of nasty bugs that can lurk in food. That's why it works as a preservative. If I told you I knew of a cheap, tasty way to kill bacteria in food before it gets to your stomach, you'd want to use it, wouldn't you? Just pass the salt (judiciously).

The more meat you eat, the more salt you'll get in the food itself. But the more fruits and vegetables you eat, the more potassium you'll get, potentially upsetting the body's balance between sodium (salt) and potassium. Furthermore, processed foods are crammed with salt, making the average American diet very high in sodium. When you cut those out, give the salt shaker a place of honor on your table. The healthier your diet is overall, the more likely you are to actually need salt!

Anyone with a tendency toward low blood pressure, fatigue, and/or "postural hypotension" (feeling dizzy when you stand up from sitting or lying down) should think about adding salt to their diet. Also, if you have problems with your adrenal hormones, your salt/potassium balance might be off. Adrenal hormones maintain the salt balance, and if they aren't fully on the job, your body may have trouble retaining salt.

now and then without any negative effect. In the middle of a crisis, reaching for a plate of cookies or a large order of fries will just make matters worse. But from a serene and stable state, a slice of Aunt Agatha's birthday cake will be a simple pleasure, not a trigger to a downward spiral.

We're Not in Eden Anymore

In an idyllic world, we might dine primarily on the fruits we pluck from the trees growing wild around us, and the seasonal produce we grow ourselves. But realistically, we are far, far from that sort of Eden. In the modern world, it is next to impossible to eat perfectly. It's hard enough to eat well. Even if you were to grow and prepare all your food yourself, eschewing the "whites" for all time, you'd still be up against soil depleted of many nutrients and foods that, as a result, aren't all they can be. For those of us who live in the real world, with ordinary human desires, it only gets more complicated from there.

Rather than further endangering our health by stressing out over standards we can't meet, we have a simple solution: nutritional therapy. Supplements can restore what's been depleted, rebuild what's damaged, and compensate for what's missing. Optimal results come from the combination of supplementation and a wholesome diet, but you don't have to eat perfectly to benefit.

Try getting everything you need out of your food. Usually, when you're feeling healthy and well and eating right most of the time, that's all you need to do. But for times when your diet is less than ideal, or when you're under excessive stress, or whenever your mood or health has slipped, supplements can restore balance and wellness.

No matter what your type, if you're "in trouble," chances are you've strayed from eating mostly natural foods. As long as you are on a natural diet, you should feel good. The well-nourished human being functions smoothly, feels good, feels optimistic, and believes wholeheartedly that it is a wonderful thing to be alive. On a natural diet, you should feel thoroughly well. If you're not, there may be external circumstances contributing to it, but you're also probably getting too much refined sugar and flour, or too much rich food, or too much junk food, and the lack of sound nutrition is creating vitamin deficiencies and chemical imbalances.

There are two ways to deal with that. One is prevention—eating better so you don't get to that point in the first place. The other (recognizing that we're all human) is treatment, or taking vitamins and supplements to help balance you out. When you're feeling blue, fatigued, or anxious, that is the time to think about supplements, which are the quickest way to eliminate the deficiencies created by careless eating.

Daily Supplements for All Types

No matter what your type, it pays to remember your ABCs: the most basic supplement program should include—for everyone—vitamins A, B, C, D—and E for good nutrition. (If the daily-supplements list for your type gives a different dosage, follow that recommendation over this one.)

Vitamin A: 15,000 IU daily from natural fish-liver oil

B vitamins: One balanced B-50 complex (50 mg doses of each B vitamin) daily; 400 mcg–1 mg folic acid daily; 100–1,000 mcg B12 daily

Vitamin C: 500–3,000 mg daily

Vitamin D: You'll get some from the fish-liver oil, and your body will make what you need from cholesterol in your skin as long as you get some sun exposure most days.

Vitamin E: 200–400 IU daily of natural mixed tocopherols from vegetable oil

---

It's Not Just *What* You Eat . . .

How you eat is just as important as *what* you eat. Take a lesson from the French. Take a lot of time for a meal—at least half an hour. Eat in a calm state of mind, in relaxed surroundings. When you are nervous or tense, your digestive system won't work properly. Don't distract yourself by reading the paper or watching television—you might forget to chew! Don't discuss unpleasant things—it is better to engage in light conversation with others or sit quietly by yourself. Studies show that if you eat in negative circumstances, you actually do not gain as much nutritive value from the food. We can improve the nutrition of anything by simply modifying the *way* in which we eat it.

Be aware of the eating process. Don't gulp your food. Chew it thoroughly before swallowing. Your saliva, which is full of digestive enzymes, has now done 50 percent of the digestion of that food, as it was designed to, *before* the food ever reaches your stomach. This is especially important as you get older, because the stomach and pancreatic digestive enzymes decline (at least, they do on the typical Western diet). If you have a lot of gas, bloating, or belching after eating, you are probably eating faster than your body can handle. In that case, your stools are likely to be poorly formed. If chewing more thoroughly doesn't result in well-formed stools, then consider taking stomach and pancreatic enzymes and reducing or eliminating coffee, tea, and other stimulants, which interfere with digestion.

When you chew slowly and give the meal your undivided attention, you are escaping for at least thirty minutes from all the tension and disease-inducing hurry and worry of your day.

Body chemistry creates brain chemistry. But it's a two-way street: Brain chemistry also creates body chemistry. There's a continuous feedback loop between the two. So, what you think is as important as what you eat, and to be truly healthy you must work in both arenas. At the most basic level, this means eating good foods and thinking good thoughts.

The promise of this book is that good nutrition will be enough to improve or stabilize your mood and bring overall wellness. But to optimize the benefits, you need to understand your character type and focus on the strengths while shoring up weaknesses. Used in combination, completing the two-way circuit, you'll maximize the incredible potential of your brain.

Resources

Psychiatrists

I. Michael Lesser, M.D.
2340 Parker St.
Berkeley, CA 94704
(510) 845-0700

Abram Hoffer, M.D.
2727 Quadra St., Suite 3A
Victoria, BC, Canada
V8T 4E5
(250) 386-8756

Hugh D. Riordan, M.D.
3100 North Hillside Ave.
Wichita, KS 67219
(316) 682-3100

Andrew Levinson, M.D.
2999 N.E. 191st St., Suite 905
Aventura, FL 33180
(305) 466-1100
www.vitalitywellness.com

Bradford Weeks, M.D.
P.O. Box 740
Clinton, WA 98236
(360) 341-2303
www.weeksmd.com

Hyla Cass, M.D.
Pacific Palisades, CA
(310) 459-9866
www.cassmd.com

Priscilla Slagle, M.D.
Palm Springs, CA
(800) 289-8487
www.thewayup.com

Garry M. Vickar, M.D.
1245 Graham Rd., Suite 506
St. Louis, MO 63031
(314) 837-4900

Michael Schachter, M.D.
2 Executive Blvd., Suite 202
Suffern, NY 10901
(845) 368-4700

Thomas Stone, M.D.
1374 E. 3700 N. Road
Kempton, IL 60946
(815) 253-6332

Professional Organizations

American Academy of Anti-Aging
  Medicine
2415 North Greenview
Chicago, IL 60614
(773) 528-4333
www.worldhealth.net

Autism Research Institute
4182 Adams Avenue
San Diego, CA 92116
(619) 281-7165
www.autismresearchinstitute.com

Cancer Control Society
2043 N. Berendo St.
Los Angeles, CA 90027
(323) 663-7801
www.cancercontrolsociety.com
Information on alternative therapies
and nutritional approaches to cancer
and other diseases

Center for Nutritional Research
P.O. Box 2620
Cottonwood, AZ 86326
(801) 264-5504
www.icnr.org

International Society of Orthomolecular Medicine
16 Florence Avenue
Toronto, Ontario, Canada
M2N 1E9
(416) 733-2117
www.orthomed.com

Nutritional Medicine
2340 Parker Street
Berkeley, CA 94704
(510) 845-0700
www.nutritionvitamintherapy.com
www.thebrainchemistrydiet.com
www.brainchemistrydiet.com

Vitamin, Food Supplement, and Instrument Suppliers To Health-Care Professionals

(Some of these vendors also serve the general public.)

ABCO Incorporated
2450 South Watney Way
Fairfield, CA 94533
(800) 678-2226
www.abcolabs.com
Food supplement and vitamin manufacturer

Allergy Research Group/
  Nutricology, Inc.
30806 Santana Street
Hayward, CA 94544
(800) 545-9960
www.nutricology.com
Nutritional supplement manufacturer/
supplier

Alternative Medicine
1650 Tiburon Blvd.
Tiburon, CA 94920
(800) 333-HEAL
www.alternativemedicine.com
Consumer periodical

AMARC
PMB 281, 539 Telegraph Cny. Rd.
Chula Vista, CA 91910
(619) 656-1980
www.polymva.net

American BioSciences
560 Bradley Parkway, Unit 4
Blauvelt, NY 10913
(888) 884-7770
www.americanbiosciences.com
Manufacturer of ImmPower

B & L Healthcare Corp.
3525 Mt. Davidson
San Jose, CA 95124
(408) 559-3008
Sells medical and dental products and
natural foods to medically ill

Natural Pages
City Spirit Publications
P.O. Box 267
Lagunitas, CA 94938
(800) 486-4794
www.naturalpages.com

Bio Meridian
12411 South 265 West, Suite F
Draper, Utah 84020
(888) 765-4665
www.biomeridian.com
Medical company selling to licensed
health-care practitioners

Bio-Tech Pharmacal, Inc.
P.O. Box 1992
Fayetteville, Arkansas 72702
(800) 345-1199
www.bio-tech-pharm.com

Licensed nutraceutical/pharmaceutical
facility

BioVitale
18218 McDurmott East, Suite C
Irvine, CA 92614
(877) 891-3395
www.biovitale.com
Structured water and nutritional supplements

Carlson Labs
15 College Drive
Arlington Heights, IL 60004
(847) 255-1600
www.carlsonlabs.com
Manufactures and distributes vitamins
and food supplements

Clarus Products International
1330 Lincoln Avenue, Suite 210
San Rafael, CA 94901
(888) 387-5956
www.clarus.com
Sells QLink pendants

College Pharmacy
3505 Austin Bluffs Pkwy, Suite 101
Colorado Springs, CO 80918
(800) 888-9358
www.collegepharmacy.com
Compounding pharmacy

Cutting Edge
P.O. Box 5034
Southampton, NY 11969
(800) 497-9516
www.cutcat.com
Products to protect the immune system
from environmental stress

Dietetics Pharma International
7599 Redwood Boulevard, Suite 214
Novato, CA 94945
(415) 892-5988
www.dieteticspharma.com
Dietary supplement distributor

Dolisos
3014 Rigel Avenue
Las Vegas, NV 89102
(800) 365-4767
Manufactures and distributes wholesale
and retail natural homeopathic remedies

Douglas Laboratories
600 Boyce Road
Pittsburgh, PA 15205
(412) 494-0122
www.douglaslabs.com
Manufactures and distributes dietary
supplements sold exclusively through
physicians

Ecological Formulas
1061B Shary Circle
Concord, CA 94518
(800) 888-4585
Distributes vitamin supplements to
health-food stores, physicians, and the
general public

Emerson Ecologics
7 Commerce Drive
Bedford, NH 03110
(800) 654-4432
www.emersonecologics.com
Distributes nutritional supplements to
health-care professionals and their
patients

Extreme Health
P.O. Box 128
Alamo, CA 94507
www.extremehealthusa.com
(800) 800-1285
Distributes oral chelation, a formula for
heavy metal toxicity

For Your Health, Inc.
13758 Lake City Way, NE
Seattle, WA 98125
(800) 456-4325
www.fyh.com
Worldwide distributor of high-quality
nutritional supplements and health aids

Freeda Vitamins
36 East 41st Street
New York, NY 10017
(800) 777-3737
www.freedavitamins.com
Prime holistic manufacturer of a
complete line of sugar-free, gluten-free,
yeast-free, kosher, and vegetarian
nutrients

Future Medical Group
(800) 882-9577
www.coralcalciumonline.com
Sells Coral calcium and vitamins
wholesale and retail

Haelan Products, Inc.
18568 142nd Avenue NE, Building F
Woodinville, WA 98072
(800) 542-3526
www.haelanproducts.com
Sells quality nutritional supplements

Heart Rhythm Instruments, Inc.
173 Essex Avenue
Metuchen, NJ 08840
(732) 635-9100
www.nervexpress.com
Quantitative assessment of autonomic
function based on heart rate variability
analysis

HOC Progressive Medical Centers
Unit 621 P.O. Box 8000
Abbots Fong, BC, Canada
V25 6H1
(888) 881-2284
www.hochealth.com
Brain injury treatment center focusing
on hyperbaric oxygen therapy

Human Alchemy/Royal Bodycare
P.O. Box 21617
Oakland, CA 94620-1617
(800) 783-0453
www.rbcglobenet.com/humanalchemy.asp

Hyssop Enterprises
7095 Hollywood Boulevard #713
Hollywood, CA 90028
(800) 228-4425
www.hyssopherb.com
Sells Hyssop products

Hickey Chemists
888 Second Avenue
New York, NY 10017
(800) 724-5566
Compounding pharmacy that provides
nutritional support to medical professionals and their clients

Ion & Light Company
2263½ Sacramento Street
San Francisco, CA 94115
(800) 426-1110
www.ionlight.com

Jarrow Formulas
1824 S. Robertson Blvd.
Los Angeles, CA 90035
(800) 726-0886
www.jarrow.com
Formulator and wholesaler of high-
quality nutritional supplements for
health-care professionals and health-
food retailers

JHS Natural Products
P.O. Box 50398
Eugene, OR 97405
(888) 330-4691
www.jhspro.com
Distributes quality medicinal mushroom extracts

Juice Plus/ NSA, Inc.
4260 East Raines Road
Memphis, TN 38118
(901) 366-9288
www.juiceplus.com
Concentrated fruit and vegetable juice
powder, enzyme active, phytonutrient
packed

Lane Labs
25 Commerce Drive
Allendale, NJ 07401
(800) 526-3005
www.lanelabs.com
Manufactures proprietary natural
supplements, available through health-
care professionals and health-food stores

Low Level Lasers, Inc.
P.O. Box 9639
Rapid City, SD 57709
(877) 862-5669
Sells low level lasers for pain control
and inflammation; class one FDA

Lipogen Products Ltd.
60 Harofeh Street
Haifa, Israel 31076
011 (972) 52 522355
www.lipogen.co.il/
Distributor and manufacturer of phos-
phatidylserine (ps)

Magnetico
5421-11th Street NE #109
Calgary, Alberta, Canada
T2E 6M4
(800) 265-1119
www.magneticosleep.com
Manufactures retail and wholesale
magnetic sleep pads

Maitake Products, Inc.
222 Bergen Turnpike
Ridgefield Park, NJ 07660
(800) 747-7418
www.maitake.com
Manufactures and sells maitake-D
fraction mushroom extract

McGuff Co., Inc.
3524 Lake Center Drive
Santa Ana, CA 92704
(800) 854-7220
Pharmaceutical distributor to health-
care professionals

Medica
702 Russell Avenue, Suite 100
Gaithersburg, MD 20877
(888) 926-6099
www.medica-usa.com
Sells and implements wellness centers

Medical Research Institute
1001 Bayhill Drive, Suite 204
San Bruno, CA 94066
(888) 448-4246
www.glucotize.com
Source for alpha lipoic acid

Metabolic Maintenance
68994 North Pine Street, Box 3600
Sisters, OR 97759
(800) 772-7873
www.metabolicmaintenance.com
Manufacturer of pure encapsulated
physician-exclusive nutritional supplements

Metagenics, Inc.
100 Avenida la Pata
San Clemente, CA 92673
(800) 692-9400
www.metagenics.com
Sells medical foods and nutritional
supplements to health-care professionals

NF Formulas
9775 SW Commerce Circle, Suite C-5
Wilsonville, OR 97070
(800) 547-4891

Nordic Naturals
5A Hangar Way
Watsonville, CA 95076
(800) 662-2544
www.nordicnaturals.com
Quality Omega-3, Omega-6 fatty acids
specialist

Novus Optimum
P.O. Box 640588
San Francisco, CA 94164
(888) 499-9100
Sells dietary supplements to enhance
brain function

Novus Research Inc.
745 N. Gilbert Road, Suite 124-223
Gilbert, AZ 85234
(800) 244-2438
www.brainlightning.com
Offers quality neurological nutrient
supplements

Nu Start, Inc.
618 Commercial Avenue
Cairo, IL 62914
(800) 246-3737
Manufacturer, distributor, and wholesale and retail seller of alternative medical instruments; ozone generator

Nutrabalance
c/o Total Health Enterprises
4730 Table Mesa Drive, Suite A2
Boulder, CO 80303
(800) 468-7903
www.nutrabalance.com
Sells software that summarizes lab data
and that provides dietary and nutritional recommendations

Orthomolecular Products, Inc.
3017 Business Park Drive
Stevens Point, WI 54481
(800) 332-2351
Sells to licensed health-care professionals

Physiologics
10701 Melody Drive, Suite 515
Northglen, CO 80234
(800) 765-6775
www.physiologics.com
Quality nutritional supplements for
health-care professionals and pharmacies

Premier Micronutrients
570B Canyon Oaks Drive
Oakland, CA 94605
(888) 606-8883
www.premiermicronutrients.com
Sells individually customized nutrients
through health-care professionals;
collects data on their efficacy

Pure Body Institute
230 South Olive Street
Ventura, CA 93001
(800) 952-7873
Herbal supplements for body and colon
cleansing and detoxification, liver
detoxification, and parasite detoxification

SCS Intensive Nutrition
1972 Republic Avenue
San Leandro, CA 94577
(800) 333-7414
www.intensivenutrition.com
Manufactures and sells high-quality
dietary supplements

Solanova
7110 Redwood Boulevard
Novato, CA 94945
(800) 200-0456
www.solanova.com
Bioavailable nutritional supplements

Symbiotics
2301 W. Hwy. 89A, Suite 107
Sedona, AZ 86336
(800) 784-4355
www.symbiotics.com
Produces and sells colostrum wholesale
to health-food stores and physicians

Tachyon Energy Research, Inc.
4400 186th Street
Redondo Beach, CA 90278
(800) 888-2509
www.takionic.com
Sells materials that attract tachyon
energy, aiding in restoring homeostasis

Thorne Research, Inc.
P.O. Box 25
Dover, ID 83825
(800) 228-1966
www.thorne.com
Sells nutritional supplements of their
own research and manufacture to
health-care professionals

Vital Nutrients
50 Silver Street
Middletown, CT 06457
(888) 328-9992
Independent lab-tested nutrients; Sells
to health-care practitioners

Vitamin Research Products
3579 Highway 50 East
Carson City, NV 89701
(800) 877-2447
www.vrp.com
Manufactures and sells pharmaceutical-
grade nutrition supplies

Willner Chemists
100 Park Avenue
New York, NY 10017
(800) 633-1106
www.willner.com

Young Living Essential Oils
1862 Anthony Court
Mountain View, CA 94040
(800) 645-7991
www.yourhealthierchoice.com
Grade A aromatherapeutic essential oils

Laboratories

Most of the tests discussed in *The Brain Chemistry Diet* can be performed by any regular laboratory. The following list of laboratories is for more extensive specialized testing in brain (and body) chemistry.

AAL Reference Laboratories, Inc.
1715 E. Wilshire #715
Santa Ana, CA 92705
(800) 522-2611
www.antibodyassay.com

Doctor's Data, Inc.
3755 Illinois Avenue
St. Charles, IL 60174
(800) 323-2784
www.doctorsdata.com

Great Plains Laboratory
11813 West 77th
Lenexa, KS 66214
(913) 341-8949
www.greatplainslaboratory.com

Great Smokies Diagnostic Laboratory
63 Zillicoa Street
Asheville, NC 28801
(800) 522-4762
www.gsdl.com

Immunosciences Lab, Inc.
8693 Wilshire Blvd., Suite 200
Beverly Hills, CA 90211
(800) 950-4686
www.immuno-sci-lab.com

International Center for Metabolic
 Testing
1305 Richmond Road
Ottawa, Ontario, Canada
K2B 7Y4
(888) 591-4124
www.icmt.com

Intracellular Diagnostics, Inc.
533 Pilgrim Drive, Suite B
Foster City, CA 94404
(800) 874-4804
www.exatest.com

MetaMetrix Clinical Laboratory
4855 Peachtree Industrial Boulevard,
Suite 201
Norcross, GA 30092
(800) 221-4640
www.metametrix.com

King James Medical Laboratory
24700 Center Ridge Road #113
Cleveland, OH 44145-5606
(800) 437-1404
www.kingjamesomegatech-lab.com

Vitamin Diagnostics
Route 35 and Industrial Road
Cliffwood Beach, NJ 07735
(732) 583-7773

US BioTek Laboratories
13758 Lake City Way NE
Seattle, WA 98125
(877) 318-8728
www.usbiotek.com

Index